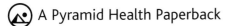
A Pyramid Health Paperback

Firm abs
flat tummy

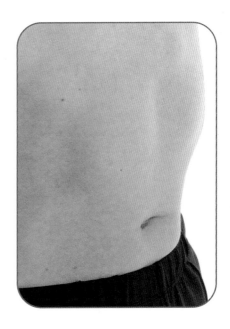

An Hachette UK Company
www.hachette.co.uk

A Pyramid Paperback

First published in Great Britain in 2009 by
Hamlyn, a division of Octopus Publishing Group Ltd
Endeavour House, 189 Shaftesbury Avenue, London WC2H 8JY
www.octopusbooks.co.uk
www.octopusbooksusa.com

Copyright © Octopus Publishing Group Limited 2009

Distributed in the U.S. and Canada by Octopus Books USA:
c/o Hachette Book Group USA
237 Park Avenue
New York NY 10017

This material was previously published as *Firm Abs Flat Stomach*.

Anne-Marie Millard asserts the
moral right to be identified
as the author of this work

ISBN 978-0-600-61803-4

A CIP catalogue record for this book is available from the
British Library

Printed and bound in China

10 9 8 7 6 5 4 3 2 1

Caution
It is advisable to check with your doctor before embarking on
any exercise programme. A doctor should be consulted on all
matters relating to health and particularly in respect of
pregnancy and any symptoms that may require diagnosis or
medical attention. While the advice and information given in
this book are believed to be accurate and the instructions given
have been devised to avoid strain, neither the author nor the
publisher can accept any legal responsibility for any injury
sustained while following the exercises.

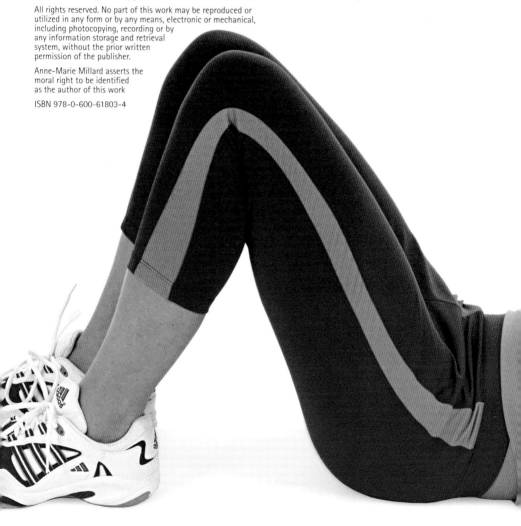

A Pyramid Health Paperback

hamlyn

Firm abs
flat tummy

Anne-Marie Millard

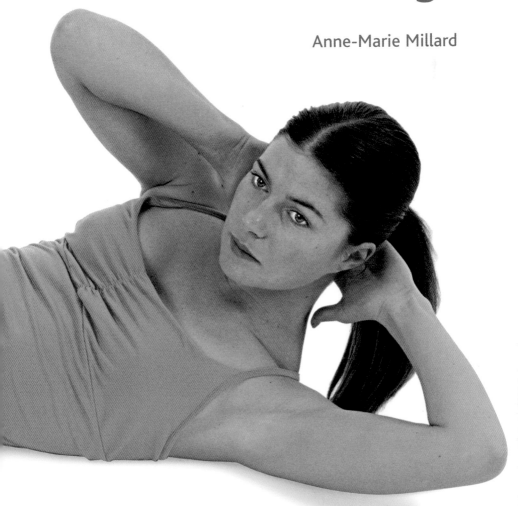

Contents

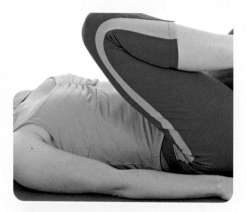

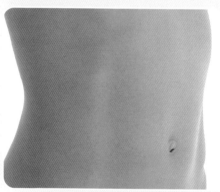

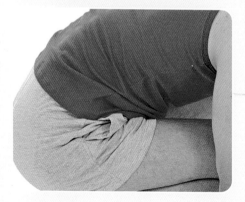

Contents

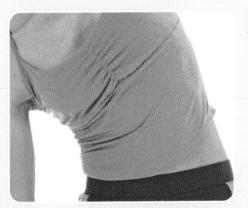

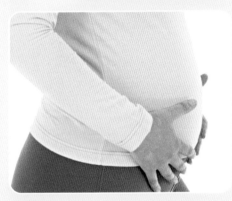

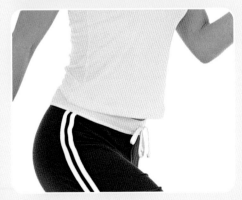

Introduction

Good news! By following a day-by-day exercise plan and combining it with healthy eating, you can achieve a flatter stomach in a month.

As you follow the 30-Day Stomach-Toning Programme in this book, you will not only get a flat stomach and firm abdominals, but you will also achieve long-lasting fitness and an overall loss of inches. What's more, as your fitness levels improve, your body will increase its ability to burn calories on a daily basis. You will learn a wide range of new exercises that you can easily fit into your daily routine.

Before starting on this or any exercise programme it is important to be clear about what you wish to achieve and how you are going to go about it. Because planning ahead is the most important part of any exercise programme, this is what the early chapters of this book are about.

Working Out Your Goals (see pages 8–21) answers some of the most common questions about health and fitness, aiming to give you an understanding of both the physiological and psychological aspects behind a successful toning and weight-loss programme. It explains the importance of working out your goals and focusing on what you want to achieve.

Focus on Diet (see pages 22–31) deals with food and why a sensible diet is so important. There are guidelines for healthy eating, as well as help to adjust your daily intake of calories, both during the programme and for life.

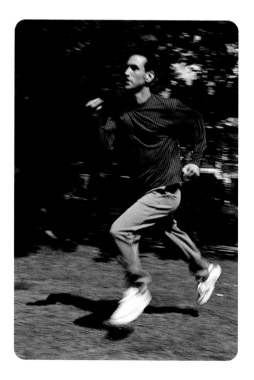

THE EXERCISES

The second part of the book contains the exercises. The **30-Day Stomach-Toning Programme** (see pages 32–105) is a comprehensive abdominal-toning programme that helps you build muscle tone and shape your midriff. It assumes you are beginning from a position of relative unfitness and each day is progressively more challenging. The tasks for each day are clearly explained and illustrated, with Tips and Technique Points to help you.

To ensure a balance between weight loss and improved general fitness and toning, the daily routine alternates between aerobic exercises (to burn calories) and resistance exercises (to tone muscles). It is not all work, however, as three rest days at intervals during the programme give you time to recuperate and renew your energy for the next stage.

Although there is cause for celebration on completion of the programme, keeping up with good eating habits and regular exercise is crucial. **Keeping Your New Body Shape** (see pages 106–115) gives advice on healthy eating and continued exercise to help you keep your new body shape.

Anyone thinking of becoming pregnant, or who has had a baby already, will know that the state of their stomach muscles can be a real worry. **Pre- and Post-Natal Exercises** (see pages 116–125) deals with how to exercise this area safely during pregnancy and ease back into exercise after delivery.

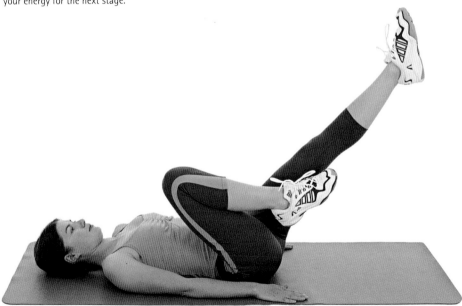

Working Out Your Goals

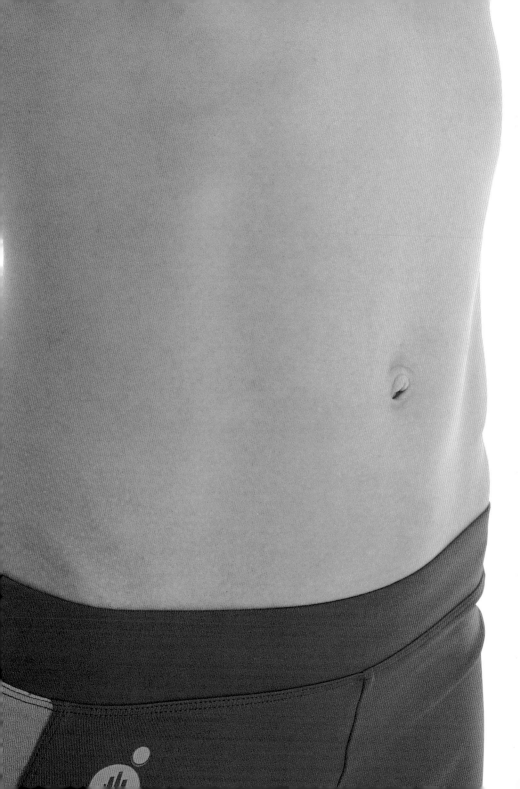

What Is Body Fat?

Body fat is the tissue in and around muscles that is made up of fat cells. Fat 'burns' very slowly to sustain the body when food is scarce. For most of us food is rarely scarce, so it has become common for many people to carry excess body fat. There is an unfortunate misconception that all body fat is bad. This is simply not true – the body needs essential fat to cushion internal organs, provide warmth and allow us to store energy for later use. It is only the excess fat that is unnecessary and can lead to long-term health problems.

Women generally carry more fat than men. This is largely to facilitate childbearing: even if a woman is starving, she should still have enough fat stored to maintain a pregnancy. If a woman's fat supplies fall dangerously low (from excessive dieting or severe illness) it is likely that her periods will stop, making it impossible to conceive. Normal, or accepted, body-fat supplies are typically between 20 and 25 per cent of overall weight for women and between 13 and 18 per cent for men.

Thanks to this support system, one of the last places these fat stores are shifted from is the area surrounding women's reproductive systems – namely the hips and stomach. Of course, this is usually the place from where most women want to lose that extra roll of flesh.

MAINTAINING A BALANCE

It is simple to understand exactly why we put on extra weight. Every individual needs a specific daily calorie intake in order to remain healthy and energized. This intake is determined by a person's Basic Metabolic Rate (BMR) (see page 30).

If you exceed your daily calorie intake by 'over-eating', the excess calories are stored in the body as fat cells in the adipose tissue, just beneath the skin. As this excess 'energy' is retained as body fat, the cells that hold the fat expand. When they become full, the cells divide to form new fat cells ready to be filled. These cells, once created, never go away. However, as long as these cells are not filled with excess fat, the body is going to look sleek and toned. What better incentive to follow a long-term healthy eating and exercise plan?

WEIGHT VS BODY FAT

It is important to realize that having 'excess fat' is not something that can be determined by how much you weigh. For example, two women of the same height and build may weigh the same, but one can look toned and slim while the other appears flabby. This is because muscle can weigh up to three times as much as fat.

When they begin an exercise programme a lot of people are distressed to find that they do not lose any weight on the scales. As they become fitter, their body fat percentage lowers and they gain lean muscle tissue (losing wobbly bits and gaining a sleek toned body on the way). Since the lean muscle weighs more than fat, they get slimmer but not necessarily lighter.

CHECKING FOR EXCESS FAT

Setting realistic goals is very important in any weight-loss programme. As you start, it is helpful to know how much excess fat you are carrying. While exercise can do wonders to get rid of unwanted pounds and help to give you a flat stomach, it can't turn a naturally short stocky person into a willowy supermodel-shape.

Be realistic and set your sights on achievable changes. An important tip before you start is to measure yourself using a tape measure, and to do so again at intervals in the programme. Fill in the Body Measurements Chart provided at the end of this chapter to plot your progress (see page 21).

There are two ways you can roughly calculate your body fat. Body Mass Index (BMI), which indicates whether you are within a normal weight range for your height, and Hip-to-Waist ratio.

CALCULATING YOUR BMI

To calculate your BMI, follow this formula:

$$BMI = \frac{weight\ (kg)}{height\ (m) \times height\ (m)}$$

If, for example, you are 1.6 m tall and weigh 65 kg, the calculation will be as follows:

$$\frac{65}{2.56} = 25.39$$

BMI RANGES

Lower than 18.5	Underweight
18.5–24.9	Normal
25–29.9	Overweight
30 and higher	Obese

CALCULATING YOUR HIP-TO-WAIST RATIO

1 Take a tape measure and measure your waist. Your waistline runs approximately around where your navel is. Pull the tape so that it fits snugly around your bare skin. Note the measurement in centimetres.

2 To measure your hips, bend your knees slightly and wrap the tape measure snugly around where the tops of the thighs meet the hips – where you bend naturally. Note the measurement in centimetres.

3 Calculate the ratio by dividing your waist measurement by your hip measurement. For example, if your waist measures 69 cm and your hips 91 cm, your hip-to-waist ratio is 0.76 (69 ÷ 91).

HIP-TO-WAIST RATIO

Women	**0.85** or less.
Men	**0.95** or less.

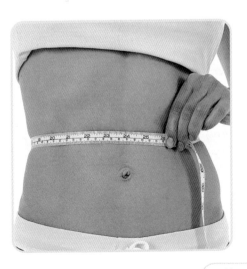

HOW TO LOSE BODY FAT

You cannot 'spot-reduce' fat. However, an added bonus of the 30-Day Stomach-Toning programme is that you can expect an overall loss of inches by the time you've finished.

Losing excess body fat is actually very simple as all you need to do is the following:

Eat Less: This does not mean going on a severe crash diet, a route that leads to more problems. Follow the guidelines given in the next chapter, Focus on Diet (see pages 22–31) to help make the correct food choices, not just for this 30-day programme but for healthy long-term living.

Exercise More: This helps the body to burn off any excess fat in the form of calories and also by replacing excess fat with lean muscle tissue, which in turn helps to increase your Basic Metabolic Rate (BMR, see page 30).

Regular exercise also:

- Increases heart and lung strength.
- Improves posture.
- Gives you more energy.
- Fosters the feel-good factor.
- Increases muscle mass.

These two principles are the key to what makes this 30-day programme so effective. Combining extra aerobic energy and an abdominal toning programme with a healthy diet not only gives you a short-term solution but helps you move forward to a much healthier and fitter life in general.

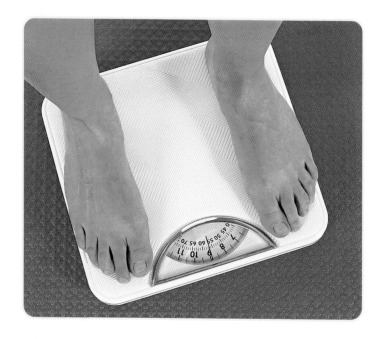

DIFFERENT BODY TYPES

Most of us inherited our body type from the family's gene pool. This means that if your mother put on fat around her mid-section it is likely that you will too. Even though body types are not scientifically defined, and many people are a combination of two, they can help you understand exactly where you are coming from and help you define your future goals.

Mesomorph

People with this body type tend to be big-boned with a strong muscular physique. Shoulders are strong, waist is narrow and posture is good. Mesomorphs can look rectangular-shaped and, fortunately for them, both losing and gaining weight are quite easy. Good mesomorph exercises include walking and short-distance running, martial arts or sports requiring balance, power and agility.

Ectomorph

People of this type are tall, with long slender necks, and lightly muscled with narrow shoulders, chests and hips. Having long limbs and small wrists and ankles, they could be described as delicate looking. With a naturally high metabolism, ectomorphs find it difficult to gain muscle and fat. This makes them a poor candidate for swimming but good at jogging, skipping, tennis and other racquet sports.

Endomorph

Endomorphs are round or soft-looking, prone to being chubby. Broader at the hips than the shoulders and small-boned, they are not naturally muscular and can carry a higher-than-average amount of body fat. With a slower metabolism than both mesomorphs and ectomorphs, endomorphs find losing weight difficult, which can in turn hide muscle tone. They are poor candidates for jogging or any high-impact activity, but can be excellent at any low-impact exercise such as walking, cycling or swimming.

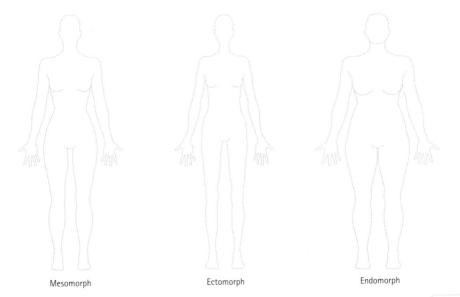

Mesomorph   Ectomorph   Endomorph

The Abdominal Muscles

Before you embark on any specific stomach-toning exercise, it is very important to understand exactly what your stomach muscles are designed to do. They flex and rotate the trunk of your body and pressurize your abdomen for normal body actions like coughing.

There are four main muscle groups involved, all of which move the body in a slightly different way. Effective abdominal toning depends on understanding exactly where each of these muscles lies, what their function involves and how to engage them.

Remember that no individual muscle works in isolation. It is only by working a combination of muscle groups that you will develop a firm and flat stomach.

CORE STABILIZATION

The ultimate aim of core stabilization (also known as core stability training) is to ensure that the deep trunk muscles are working correctly. These control and protect the lumbar spine (the five vertebrae lying between the lowest ribs and the hips) during dynamic movements, such as lifting heavy boxes, running or weight training.

We begin this core stability work by learning to contract the transverse abdominus (and multifidus) muscles safely and effectively. It is very important that you get into the correct starting position for this exercise – namely, into a 'neutral spine' position.

This simply means that while you are lying on the floor with your knees bent, about to perform a basic sit-up, your lumbar spine should neither be arched up nor flattened against the floor, but aligned naturally with a small gap between the floor and your back.

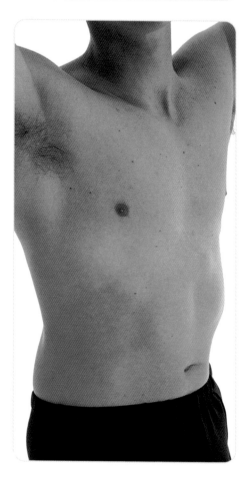

THE MUSCLE GROUPS

Transversus Abdominis

Of the four front muscles, this one lies closest to your internal organs until it crosses under your navel. Below the navel, the lower fibres of this broad, flat, horizontal muscle form a sheath opening with two other muscles, which permits the rectus abdominis to push through and attach securely to the pubis bone. As the transversus abdominis contracts, it compresses the internal organs, which helps the lungs to exhale and the body to perform the normal process of elimination. These are the muscles you work when you hold your stomach in – they are an essential element in your abdominal resistance programme.

Internal Obliques

These two muscles lie on top of the transversus abdominis, one on each side. The muscle fibres start at the hip and run diagonally upward to meet the lower ribs and diagonally downward to the groin. Lateral flexion and torso rotation to the same side are the main functions of these muscles. These muscles are involved in the Side Bend exercises (see page 50).

External Obliques

These wide but thin muscles originate at the border of the lower ribs and extend forwards and down. The fibres run at right angles to those of the internal obliques. The primary functions of these muscles are to bend the spine to the same side and rotate the torso to the opposite side. These are the muscles involved in waist or side exercises.

Rectus Abdominis

This outermost frontal muscle stretches vertically from the ribcage to the pubis bone. The function of the rectus abdominis is to shorten the distance between the breastbone and the pelvic girdle. If you have a small percentage of body fat and have a well-developed rectus abdominis you will have what is commonly known as a 'six-pack', namely three paired blocks of muscle on each side of the mid-line. The rectus abdominis is the main muscle worked in a Basic Sit-up (see page 51).

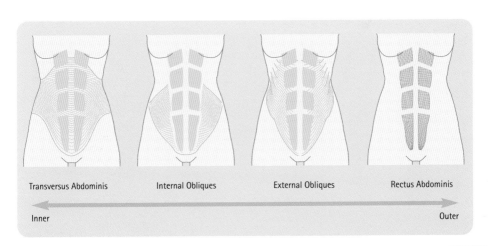

| Transversus Abdominis | Internal Obliques | External Obliques | Rectus Abdominis |

Inner → Outer

Good Posture

Good posture is the foundation stone of all your movements whether you are exercising or sitting at a desk. Poor posture can lead to incorrect body alignment (and the musculo-skeletal problems associated with it) and it can also make your stomach look fatter than it actually is!

Standing and moving correctly is down to habit. How are you sitting at the moment? Are you slouching in a chair? Are your legs crossed? Both of these positions can have a negative effect on your posture.

While it is not necessary to spend a lifetime sitting on hard high-back chairs, reminding yourself every now and then to sit and stand up straight will make a huge difference, not just to how you look but how you feel about yourself.

KYPHOSIS AND THE DOWAGER'S HUMP

Of the common postural problems, two stand out. Kyphosis, or rounded shoulders, often results from tight chest muscles, which are caused either by a particular working practice or by over-development of the pectoral (chest) muscles through exercise or sport. These tight chest muscles cause the chest to become concave and the shoulders to round forwards.

The best way to correct this fault is to stretch the chest muscles and strengthen the spinal muscles through daily posture exercises.

The second common problem – the Dowager's Hump – is caused by a poor sitting position over a period of time and is very common in office workers. The chin juts forwards and the upper spine curves to compensate. The abdominal muscles are unable to work properly and the pelvis tips backwards, resulting in a sagging appearance.

Good posture is simply about regular habit – you need to keep reminding yourself to stand correctly as it takes a conscious effort to pull yourself into alignment. Spend a few minutes each day doing the following exercises, which are designed to open, stretch and strengthen all the postural muscles.

HOW TO STAND WITH GOOD POSTURE

1 Place your weight evenly on both feet. This might sound a bit odd but most of us tend to favour one side more than the other, so spend a few seconds rocking your bodyweight from one foot to the other until you come to a rest at an even point.

2 Now extend up through the thighs and feel the pelvis rest lightly on top of the thighs. Stretch up through the spine. Let the shoulders drop naturally down and away from your ears.

3 Soften the ribcage, drawing the bottom rib down towards your hips.

4 Now tighten the abdominals, drawing the navel in towards the back of the spine.

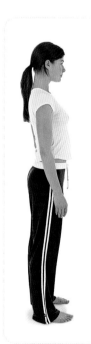

FOUR DAILY POSTURE EXERCISES

1 Lie on your back. Place your hands behind your head and press your elbows down to touch the floor.

Hold for 10 seconds

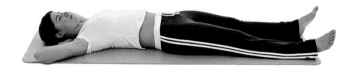

2 Sit in a chair and lean backwards. Place your hands behind your neck and press out your elbows.

Hold for 10 seconds

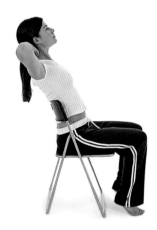

3 Lie on your stomach. Clasp your hands behind your back and raise your shoulders and chest off the floor.

Hold for 10 seconds

4 Stand with a book on your head. Feel your neck lengthening and jaw slightly tilting forwards. Lift the chest.

Hold for 10 seconds, then slowly walk around the room.

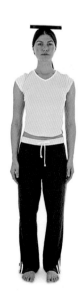

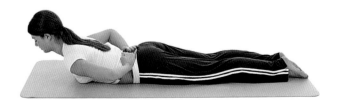

Keeping to the Programme

Keeping to the 30-day programme will be easier for some than others. We all know our individual faults and failings and should be able to predict what might go wrong and when, but – even with the best of intentions – most people are likely to encounter some blips along the way. Don't let these low points hinder your progress. The most important thing is to get back on track as soon as possible. Follow these simple tips to help keep you on the straight and narrow.

GIVE YOURSELF A REALITY CHECK

To improve your body shape successfully, you must be clear about exactly why you are doing it. There is no point even beginning this or any exercise programme if you do not believe that you can achieve your goals. There will be some days when you are not going to achieve exactly what you set out to do, but remember that this is perfectly normal, rather than thinking 'I am so useless, why did I ever think I could do it' and then abandoning all the good work you have already done.

Make sure you are doing the programme for yourself – not because a friend or partner made some cutting remark about 'the size of your belly'. This way you will be less inclined to slip back into the negative eating and non-exercise habits which you had before.

Complete your mission statement (see opposite) and keep it somewhere prominent so you will be reminded of it every day.

PLAN AHEAD

Sit down at the weekend and plan your week ahead. Enter your daily exercise routines in at a feasible time on the kitchen calendar, in a diary or a personal organizer. Then, make sure you actually do it: spend the first 7–10 days doing exactly what you planned and it will turn from being a chore to a routine. Keeping to the programme is all about habit, and these are easier to modify than you might think.

In much the same way, plan your weekly menu. Write a daily food list and buy only those foods. If you have only healthy food in the house then it is much easier to resist temptation.

ENLIST SUPPORT

Tell people what you are trying to achieve, but make sure they are the right people. Unfortunately there are some people out there who are going to have a more negative influence than a positive one – the sort who, when you have a choice between a cake and an apple, will undermine your confidence and insist you have the cake.

Choose people who are going to be genuinely pleased for you and will give you positive moral support and a boost when you feel you are slipping. Ask them to keep an eye on you and for their help. It is amazing how people's attitudes can change when they feel involved and needed. Just make sure you are surrounded by supportive people.

CONQUER THE ALL-OR-NOTHING FEAR

Accept the fact that you will have bad days. Days where you don't do any exercise or eat healthily. It is not the end of the world. Human nature is such that we are all prone to slip-ups every now and then. Just make sure you get back on track the next day. Don't

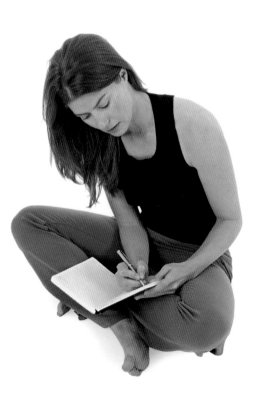

make excuses, starve yourself or do extra exercise either. This will not help. Just carry on with the plan and tell yourself it won't happen again. Start again as you mean to go on.

WRITE YOUR MISSION STATEMENT

Just buying this book means you have already started the journey towards your goal. Now is the time to personalize it. In your mission statement, set out in black and white why you have decided to exercise, what you are going to achieve, how it will change the way you look and feel and what you are going to do once you have achieved this.

One example could be 'I know I can't change my whole body, but if I can fit into my pre-pregnancy jeans then I am going to feel so much better about myself. When I do fit into them again I am going to reward myself with a shopping trip', while another might say 'Someone took a photo of me in a swimsuit last summer. I looked awful. I am determined that this year I will look better'.

Even if you think this seems a rather pointless exercise, give it a chance. It really is one of the most important things to do at the beginning of this programme. It might take a while to get it right but don't worry about feeling silly; no one else needs to read or see it, so be as honest as you can.

Once you have completed your mission statement, write it out and keep it in a place where you can read it whenever you feel your motivation failing.

Fitness Assessment

If you have doubts about your health, it is wise to consult a doctor, physiotherapist or other medical practitioner before you start this or any other exercise routine. If you answer 'yes' to any of the questions in either of the questionnaires below, then you should see a consultant.

Once you know you are in good health, use the tests opposite to establish your fitness level.

SHOULD YOU SEE A DOCTOR?

1 Have you ever been diagnosed with a heart condition, or is there any history of heart disease in your family?

2 Are you more than 19 kg (3 stone/42 lbs) overweight?

3 Do you have high blood pressure?

4 Are you diabetic?

5 Do you have asthma or a history of breathing problems?

6 Are you pregnant or trying to become pregnant?

7 Have you recently given birth?

8 Have you had surgery in the last six weeks?

9 Have you experienced chest pain during physical activity?

10 Have you ever been advised by a doctor to avoid exercise?

SHOULD YOU SEE A PHYSIOTHERAPIST?

Physiotherapists and osteopaths play an important role in the prevention of injury. It is wise to remember that prevention is better than cure.

1 Do you suffer from knee pain?

2 Have you ever had shin splints?

3 Do you suffer from lower-back problems?

4 Do you suffer twinges in your shoulders or upper back muscles?

5 Have you ever been told not to exercise for any length of time by a relevant professional?

6 Do you have bunions or other foot problems?

7 Have you ever fractured or broken any bones?

8 Have you ever had surgery on a joint or ligament?

FITNESS LEVEL

Many workouts in the programme specify a number of repetitions or a length of time to perform the exercise according to your level of fitness. Work through the following sections to determine whether you should choose Level 1 or Level 2.

Hip-to-Waist Ratio

To see which level you fall into calculate your hip-to-waist ratio (see page 11) and refer to the ranges here:

1	Women	above 0.85
	Men	above 0.95
2	Women	0.7–0.85
	Men	0.8–0.95
3	Women	below 0.7
	Men	below 0.8

1-Minute Sit-up Test

This test assesses your strength and the postural strength of your stomach muscles. Perform as many Basic Sit-ups as you can in 1 minute (see page 51). Try to use a good technique and move in a controlled way. Now compare with the scoring chart.

1 Women   24 or below
     Men   24 or below
2 Women   25–45
     Men   25–45
3 Women   46 or more
     Men   46 or more

3-Minute Step Test

This tests your cardiovascular system. Use a step, stair or a stable chair 40 cm (16 in) high and do step-ups at a rate of roughly 30 per minute for 3 minutes. Stop, take your pulse (see page 35) for 15 seconds and then multiply this figure by 4.

1 Women   167 or more
     Men   157 or more
2 Women   141–166
     Men   131–156
3 Women   140 and below
     Men   130 and below

What is Your Level?

Award yourself 1, 2 or 3 points for each test, depending on whether your score is in category 1, 2 or 3. Add up your scores. If you scored 5 or below you should choose Level 1 and if you scored 6 or above follow Level 2.

Follow the instructions for your level throughout the 30-day programme. When you have completed the programme, test your fitness level again. If you have moved up a level, you should continue at this level for the maintenance exercises (see pages 106–115).

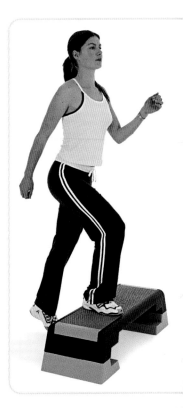

BODY MEASUREMENTS CHART

Take your measurements before you start the programme, half-way through and at the end, to see how your dimensions have changed.

	Day 1	Day 15	Day 30
Upper arm – left			
Upper arm – right			
Chest			
Waist			
Hips			
Upper thigh – left			
Upper thigh – right			

Focus
on Diet

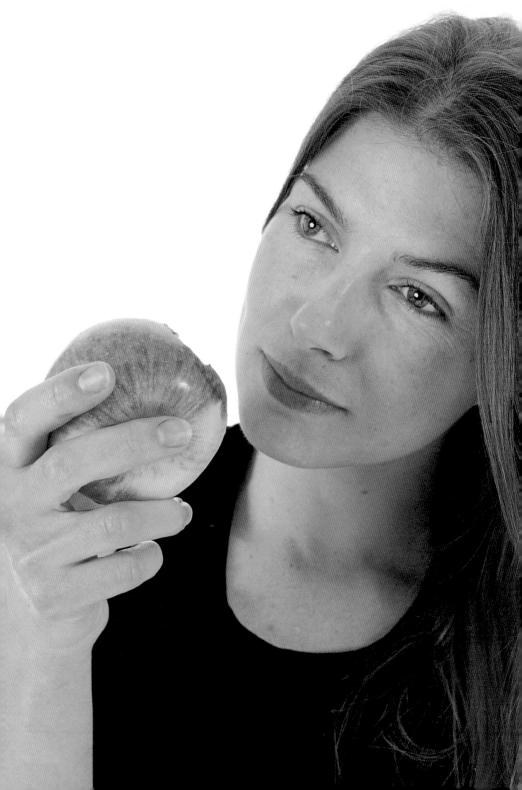

Eating Right

A healthy diet is primarily about balance. Our bodies need certain amounts of carbohydrates, proteins, fats, vitamins and minerals in order to function properly. They also need plenty of water (see page 27). Many nutritionists agree that the best long-term strategy is to eat a sensible daily diet comprising 60 per cent carbohydrates, 10 per cent protein and 30 per cent fat.

It is all too easy to neglect our diets, but it is well worth taking the time to think about what you eat, as a sensible diet will boost energy and vitality and needn't involve a lot of preparation.

CARBOHYDRATES

There are two different types of carbohydrates: simple sugars (such as sugar, jam and sweets) and complex sugars (dense starchy foods). Unfortunately, both have had a very bad press recently. In fact, complex carbohydrates in particular are vital for sensible weight loss and energized living.

The right amount of carbohydrates (combined with fat) is vital to create energy. No matter how low in intensity or aerobic the exercise, the human body cannot burn fat alone. Fat can only be used for energy alongside carbohydrates. So it is imperative to make sure that 60 per cent of your daily diet is made up of carbohydrates for you to effectively 'fat-burn'. Just make sure you are eating predominantly the right sort – eat more complex sugars and fewer simple sugars.

COMPLEX CARBOHYDRATES

The following foods contain complex carbohydrates:
- Breads
- Cereals
- Pasta
- Rice
- Starchy vegetables
- Legumes

FIBRE

Fibre is an essential element in our diets as it aids the digestive process and helps us to feel full. The best form of fibre is in wholemeal bread, while probably the most obvious fibre is found in fruit and vegetables. These also contain many other useful vitamins and minerals, as well as a high proportion of water, which again is useful for digestion. Corn, rice and pulses are also good sources of fibre.

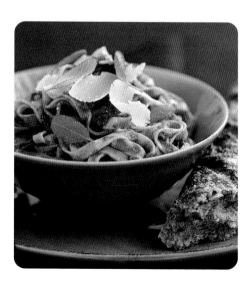

PROTEIN

The body needs protein to function healthily, but it should be limited to just 10 per cent of your daily intake of food. In recent years high protein and low carbohydrate diets have been very popular, but research has shown that the information surrounding these diets is misleading and that following them can lead to health problems. Among these are fatigue due to the loss of glycogen (a vital energy source) from the muscles; and bad breath and nausea caused by ketosis, which results because the body breaks down fat differently. Furthermore, excess protein is stored in the body as fat and can exacerbate the symptoms of both liver and kidney disease.

There is no need to worry if your protein consumption is a little higher than needed every now and again – maybe you just can't resist meat – but do be aware that if you consistently consume considerably more than 10–15 per cent of your total calorie intake as protein you could increase your health risks.

SOURCES OF PROTEIN
- Meat
- Fish
- Poultry
- Game
- Eggs
- Dairy products (such as cheese and yogurt)
- Soya
- Cereal grains (such as barley and rice)
- Vegetables (such as peas)
- Pulses

THE GLYCAEMIC INDEX

An effective way of classifying food is by the Glycaemic Index (GI). This categorizes foods by how quickly they affect the body's blood-sugar levels. Many staples of our Western diet, like potatoes, cereals and sugary foods, are high-GI, meaning they are sources of quick-release energy that fuels the body with sugar rapidly, and just as quickly leaves it craving more.

Low-GI foods are a source of slow-release energy and don't cause the energy ups and downs that make you want to snack. Here are some examples of low- and high-GI foods:

LOW-GI FOODS	HIGH-GI FOODS
Apples	Bananas
Oranges	Dried fruit
Kiwis	Watermelon
Avocados	Tomatoes
Broccoli	Parsnips
Rice noodles	Potatoes
Wholegrain bread	White bread
Wholegrain rice	White rice
Porridge	Breakfast cereals
Almonds	Cashew nuts
Brazil nuts	Rice cakes
Chickpeas	Broad beans
Lentils	Red meat
Chicken	Chicken skin
Oily fish	Battered fish
Skimmed milk	Whole milk
Soya milk	Cream
Full-fat yogurt	Low-fat yogurt
Olive oil	Butter
Herbal tea	Coffee

FAT

Contrary to popular opinion, fat is an essential part of a healthy diet. Again, it is very important that you are consuming the right sort of fat, the advice being to eat predominantly unsaturated fat. Fat is essential for many reasons:

- Protection of internal organs.
- Temperature control.
- Uptake and storage of fat-soluble vitamins.
- Energy.
- Growth, development and repair of body tissues.
- In women, storage and modification of reproductive hormones.

Fats have received a bad press because most people exceed the recommend daily intake of 30 per cent fat in their daily diet, consuming instead 40–45 per cent. These high levels dramatically increase the risk of ill health in the form of two main problems: obesity and coronary heart disease.

Like carbohydrates, fats come in two forms: saturated fats (these are mainly from animal sources and tend to be solid at room temperature) and unsaturated fats (these are mainly from plant sources and tend to be liquid at room temperature).

Try to get your fat intake in the form of 'good' (unsaturated) fat: eat oily fish (salmon and mackerel, for example) and use cold-pressed, good-quality oils for stir-frying and for dressing salad.

SOURCES OF UNSATURATED FATS:
✓ Olive oil
✓ Rapeseed oil
✓ Sunflower oil
✓ Corn oil
✓ Oily fish (such as mackerel, salmon, tuna, sardines)

SOURCES OF SATURATED FATS:
✗ Butter
✗ Cream
✗ Lard
✗ Cheese
✗ Animal fat
✗ Coconut butter
✗ Palm oil

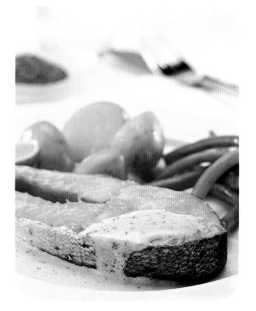

WATER

Our bodies are made up of around 60 per cent water. Besides helping to regulate body temperature, water is a solvent for the nutrients and wastes stored in your tissues, which can then be eliminated quickly and easily. We lose around 2–2.5 litres (3½–4 pints) of water a day at rest. If you are doing any exercise, this amount increases by a further 1–2 litres (1¾–3½ pints), so you will need to drink more water. Being dehydrated can slow down the metabolism and therefore energy generation, making you (and your muscles) feel tired.

Although food contains some water, most of your intake needs to be consumed separately. A good way to do this is to have a sip of water every 15 minutes or so. Remember that some drinks – coffee, tea, alcohol and many soft drinks – accelerate water loss from the body, so drink water instead.

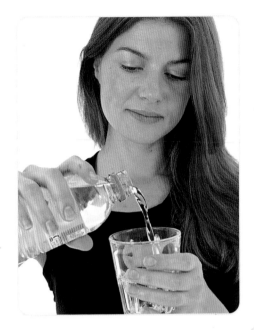

EASY STEPS TO A HEALTHIER DIET

INCREASE YOUR INTAKE OF:
✓ Fruit and vegetables
✓ Fibre-rich food (unrefined starches, fruit and vegetables)
✓ Complex carbohydrates (dense starchy foods)
✓ Water
✓ Variety in your daily diet

DECREASE YOUR INTAKE OF:
✗ Saturated fat
✗ Animal protein
✗ Sugar
✗ Salt
✗ Alcohol, fizzy drinks, coffee and tea

VITAMIN AND MINERAL SUPPLEMENTS

If you eat a healthy, balanced diet, adequate in energy and including a wide variety of foods, you should have no problem getting all the vitamins and minerals you need. Only if your diet does not provide enough vitamins and minerals and your body stores are low should you consider taking a low-dose multi-vitamin and mineral supplement. It is important not to exceed your daily requirements – more does not mean better and, in some cases, can be toxic.

THE HEALTHY EATING PYRAMID

The healthy eating pyramid translates general dietary guidelines into real food choices. This pyramid is a guide for maintaining a balanced diet, to help you not just for the 30-day programme but for life.

The food groups that make up the layers of the pyramid are arranged in order of the volume in which they should be eaten. Breads, grains and cereals – these should be eaten in the largest amounts; aim to eat a portion at each meal, about 5 servings per day. Fruit and vegetables – aim to eat 5 portions a day. Proteins – aim to eat 2–3 servings a day. Dairy products such as milk, yogurt and cheese are an important source of protein and calcium – aim to eat 2–3 servings a day. Fats, oils and sweets should be used sparingly.

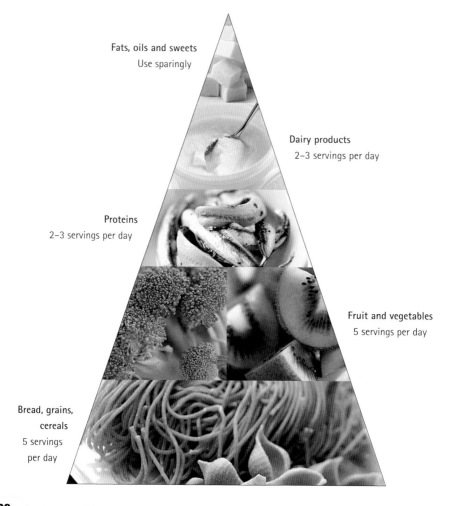

Fats, oils and sweets
Use sparingly

Dairy products
2–3 servings per day

Proteins
2–3 servings per day

Fruit and vegetables
5 servings per day

Bread, grains,
cereals
5 servings
per day

KEEP A FOOD DIARY

Whether you want to lose weight or not, it is a good idea to keep a food diary so you can assess how healthy your diet is. Write down everything you eat in the diary for the whole of the 30-day programme. Use a notebook small enough to carry around with you, but big enough to fit in the details. Write down exactly what you eat and record when and why you ate it and how you felt before, during and after eating. It is a good idea to make the entries as soon as you have eaten – it is very easy to forget snacks, but the only person you will be cheating is yourself.

If possible, begin your food diary before you start the exercise programme, even if it is only a few days before. It can be a real eye-opener to see just how much you habitually eat. After a few days of filling in the diary, you should see a pattern emerge and you will also get a good idea whether your daily diet is all you imagine it to be. Looking at the diary will show clearly where you eat any excess food. Unnecessary snacks are often the enemy in either losing fat or maintaining a steady weight.

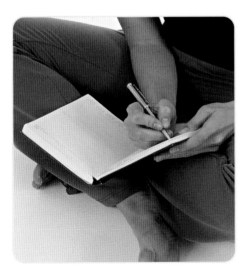

SAMPLE DAILY FOOD DIARY

Breakfast

On the train at 8.15am

- Running late so just had banana from
  fruit bowl – will grab something later

10.00am

- Really hungry and haven't time to go out
  and get something to eat. Resort to packet
  of crisps from vending machine.

Lunch

In a café at midday (early lunch because I
was really hungry)

- Baked potato with beans (no butter) –
  really did the trick: filling and delicious
- Orange and carrot juice

3.30pm

- Cup of coffee and half a bar of
  chocolate – bored and needed
  something sweet

Dinner

At home at 6.45pm

- Pasta with tomato and tuna sauce
- Small bowl of ice-cream
- Sparkling mineral water

How to Lose Weight

So many conflicting schools of thought exist about the best way to lose weight that it is no wonder that so much confusion surrounds the topic. Should you eat a protein-only diet? Live off soup? Take vitamins daily? Problems arise because many people flick from one extreme to another – fuelled by enthusiasm they starve their bodies according to the latest diet fad and end up binging guiltily. There is no need to cut out any one food group, such as carbohydrates, to lose body fat. Instead, the overall amount of food we take in needs to be reduced.

The problem for most of us is that we consume too much and our excess food intake is then stored as extra fat deposits. The solution is to know exactly what we should and shouldn't be eating and how many calories we should be consuming on an average day to make sure we can reverse or at least halt the process of accumulating extra layers of body fat.

WHAT IS METABOLISM?

There are many myths about metabolism but, simply put, it is the amount of energy required to keep the resting body provided with energy. While it is true that some people have slower metabolic rates than others, it is possible to do something about it.

One of the main influences on BMR is body composition. Even at rest, a muscle cell is metabolically more active than a fat cell. The more lean muscle (as opposed to fat) you carry, the quicker and more effective (even at rest) your metabolic rate will be. All the more reason to burn off that excess fat and replace it with lean muscle!

The higher the level of activity, the more calories need to be consumed. This is very difficult to predict, as it is not easy to measure someone's energy expenditure on the move. However, the following estimates can be used as a guide:

Sedentary lifestyle: add 20 per cent. This applies to someone who, for example, has a desk-bound job and either drives or takes public transport to work. Additional exercise during the day is minimal.

Moderately active lifestyle: add 50 per cent. This is the lifestyle of someone who walks or cycles to work, or who has an active occupation where they are on their feet all day like a teacher or a nurse. If their job

CALCULATING YOUR BMR

Your daily calorie intake can be calculated by working out your Basic Metabolic Rate (BMR), using the following formula:

25 kcals x bodyweight (in kilograms) = number of calories (kcals) you need per day.

does involve a lot of sitting, they get out and about in their breaks. In the evening they will do some formal exercise – such as aerobics classes, swimming or a game like squash or football – three or four times a week. At the weekends they may go cycling or walking.

Very active lifestyle: add 100 per cent. This describes someone who has a very active occupation, like an exercise teacher or someone who works out most days in addition to being generally very active. Of course, many people will fall somewhere between these three. Estimate your own activity levels and work out your daily calorie requirements.

HOW TO BOOST YOUR METABOLISM

In order to get the optimum boost to your metabolism, you should follow these simple rules:

Don't dramatically cut calories. A very strict diet is guaranteed to backfire. Your body is programmed to defend your normal weight, so when you severely cut your daily calorie intake to, say, less than 1,000 kcals a day, your metabolic rate adjusts to conserve the few calories you do eat.

Don't wait too long between meals. Exercise regularly and eat small frequent meals throughout the day to keep energy levels up. The bonus is that metabolizing food requires energy, so when you are eating those small frequent meals you may be burning a few extra calories too. Waiting too long between meals can also leave you vulnerable to over-eating or craving high-fat or high-sugar foods.

Don't skip breakfast. If you do, your metabolism remains slow. The whole point of breakfast is to 'break' the overnight 'fast'. Your body has been conserving energy all night long and needs a meal to jump-start its metabolism.

YOUR WEIGHT-LOSS PLAN

Healthy living and eating is your responsibility. It is you, and only you, who can turn down the offer of pudding or the second glass of wine. It is your willpower that is going to help you succeed with this 30-day plan.

It is sensible to try to lose about half a kilogram (a pound) a week, which is equivalent to 3,500 kcals. With this in mind, you should aim to cut around 500 kcals a day for the duration of the 30-day programme. This is not as stringent as it sounds and can easily be done by simply avoiding any high-fat foodstuffs, such as cakes, chocolate and crisps. You should also avoid alcoholic drinks.

REMOVING TEMPTATION

Clear your cupboards. Before you start the 30-day programme, go through all your food cupboards and give away or throw out anything you feel might trip you up over the course of the next few weeks.

Be ruthless. Leftover birthday cake? Ask your partner to take it to work. Tins of your favourite biscuits? Give them to your next-door neighbour or donate them to the local church. Not only will this clear-out leave you with less temptation but it will also set you off on a very positive mental note.

Plan your grocery shop. Decide on your menu for the week and then shop accordingly. This will help you not only to keep to the straight and narrow but also to avoid impulse purchases, saving money in the process.

Prepare ahead. Lots of dishes can be cooked in advance and then frozen, ready to be thawed at a suitable time. Make extra portions of freezer-friendly foods so you will never be caught short and have to resort to calorie-laden takeaways!

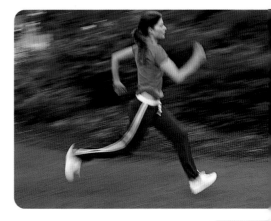

How to Lose Weight   **31**

30-Day Stomach-Toning Programme

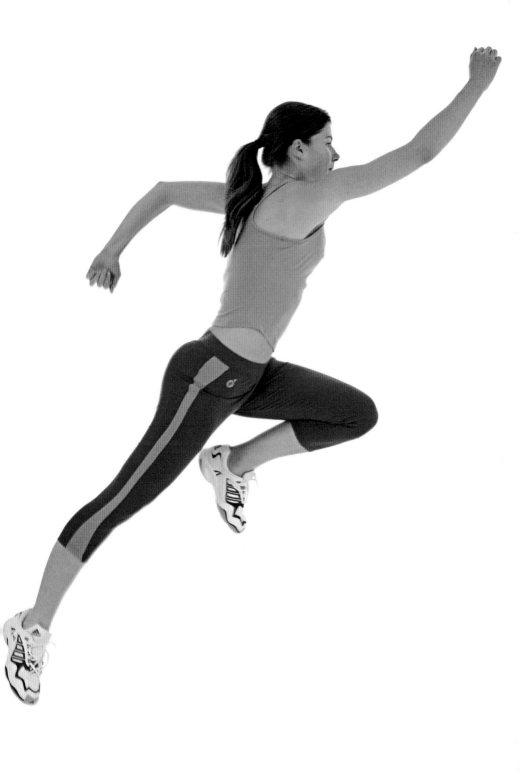

Basic Equipment

In the interests of a long-term fitness regime, it's worthwhile investing in some good-quality exercise equipment. Most of the aerobic workouts in this book, however, do offer an alternative, equipment-free workout, in case you do not wish to buy extra equipment.

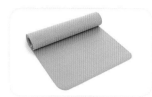

Mat: many different types of mat are available. Thickness and comfort are the main considerations on a hard floor, while on a carpet the main aim is to avoid getting the floor too sweaty. Look for a mat that is washable. Alternatively, a thick towel can be used instead.

Trampet or Rebounder: generally, the better the quality, the more stable it is. Try it first in the shop to make sure it feels sturdy enough and you feel comfortable on it, and make sure it has non-slip feet.

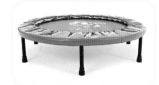

Skipping rope: choose whatever kind suits you – handles can be plastic or wooden, and ropes can be leather or synthetic – but always buy one which has adjustable rope length. (See also Day 13, pages 70–71.)

Stability ball (or 'Swiss' ball): widely available from sports shops. The size of ball varies according to your height – check the manufacturers' guidelines or the list below. Buy one that has its own pump (and keep it nearby).

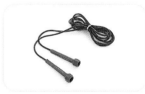

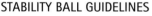

STABILITY BALL GUIDELINES

Ball Size	Your Height
45 cm (18 in) ball	below 1.5 m (5 ft) tall
55 cm (22 in) ball	1.5–1.7 m (5 ft–5 ft 7 in) tall
65 cm (26 in) ball	1.7–1.9 m (5 ft 8 in–6 ft 3 in) tall
75 cm (30 in) ball	over 1.9 m (6 ft 3 in) tall

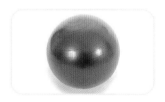

Step: invest in a good, sturdy one. Make sure it is reasonably long, is height adjustable and has a non-slip bottom and top surface. It is possible to use a house step provided it is deep enough for your whole foot to fit on.

Hand weights: weights of 2.5–4.5 kg (5–10 lb) are suitable for the exercises in this book. There are many styles available, ranging from chrome to sponge-covered, which come in a variety of weights. Most women will need to begin with a 2.5 kg (5 lb) set and possibly build up to a 4.5 kg (10 lb) set if they find their strength is increasing. Men will need to use the 4.5 kg (10 lb) set from the start.

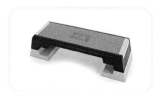

Heart-rate monitor: these range from very simple models to hi-tech ones, which allow data to be downloaded into a personal computer. They keep check on exactly how hard you are working without you needing to take your pulse. A simple model will suffice for the exercises in this book.

DETERMINING HEART RATE

To be certain you are working at your most effective rate, it is important to know your heart rate in beats per minute (BPM). Instructions for cardiovascular workouts will tell you at what percentage of your MHR (maximum heart rate) you should be working. Either take your pulse reading in the traditional way or use a heart-rate monitor, and then refer to the chart below.

Reading Your Pulse

This is an accurate and age-old way of checking you are working at the correct percentage of MHR. The only disadvantage is you have to stop exercising to do it and it can take a little practice to refine your technique. Find the pulse point at your wrist: follow the line of your thumb, then place two fingers (not your thumb) about 2.5 cm (1 in) below your wrist joint. Count the beat for 15 seconds, then multiply it by 4 to get your pulse in BPM.

Using a Heart-rate Monitor

A strap around your chest monitors your heart rate and transmits it to a watch-like device on your wrist. This is the easiest way to keep an eye on your heart rate since it gives you continuous BPM readings.

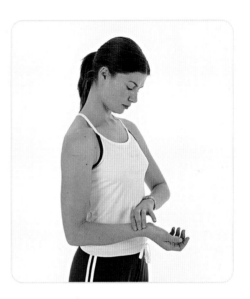

BPMS FOR DIFFERENT AGE GROUPS

Your **BPM** for any percentage of **MHR** is age-related. So, for instance, if you are aged 31–36 and the workout says work at 70 per cent MHR, your BPM should be about 130. Any higher, and you need to slow down. Any lower, and you need to up the intensity of the work.

Age	70 per cent	75 per cent	80 per cent	85 per cent	90 per cent
18–25	139	149	159	169	179
26–30	134	144	153	163	172
31–36	130	140	149	158	168
37–42	126	135	144	153	162
43–50	121	129	138	147	155
51–55	116	124	133	141	149

How and When to Exercise

When you exercise is an individual choice. It is commonly thought that the optimum time is during the afternoon. Sadly, most of us are working then, so the best option is to try out a few different times to see what suits you best.

Are you a morning person? If so, then getting up that little bit earlier to exercise won't fill you with dread. However, if you are not, then trying to commit yourself to exercising first thing is unlikely to work: you will end up dreading the idea of your workout and may give up altogether.

On the other hand, after a day of work even the idea of exercising may set you yawning. You will be surprised, however, how quickly an evening workout can re-energize you, leaving you feeling relaxed and refreshed, and free of the day's tensions.

Where to exercise is again a very personal choice. One benefit of this book is that these workouts can be done anywhere at any time. Even on holiday or staying with friends, you have no excuse. At home, choose a room with adequate space, good ventilation, a stereo or radio and, ideally, one that is reasonably private. Constant interruptions are not conducive to a decent, thorough workout.

FOLLOWING THE EXERCISES

Resistance exercises (those that tone and/or strengthen the muscles) are broken down into 'sets and repetitions'. For the body to get the optimum benefit from each exercise yet not tire too quickly, you are not expected to do all the work in one go.

If, for example, you are asked to do 2 sets of 10 repetitions (2 x 10), begin with 10 repetitions of the exercise, rest (do nothing) for 30–60 seconds to allow the working muscles to recuperate, and then perform another set of 10 repetitions. You will have done 10 repetitions, twice.

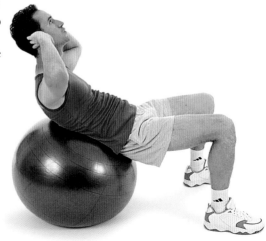

Slow and Controlled

It is very tempting to hurry through a workout to get it over with, or to fool yourself that you are working especially hard. In fact, all exercise (unless otherwise stated) should be done slowly, under control and making sure you use good technique. The Technique Points given on the exercise pages serve to make each individual exercise more effective.

Take your time with each and every move during the resistance workouts. Concentrate on what you are doing and do not let yourself become distracted. Remember that quality is always better than quantity.

Keeping Joints 'Not Locked Out'

This simply means keeping a slight bend in the joint in question so it is the muscle not the skeleton taking the strain of your workload. For example, 'do not lock out your knees' means keeping a very slight bend in your knee joint.

What to Wear?

Footwear is most important. While they needn't be too expensive, shoes must be of decent quality and fit well, and should be replaced every 640 km (400 miles) or so. Shop for shoes at the end of the day or after a workout when your feet are at their largest. Wear your usual exercise socks and do not assume that training shoes will be the same size as everyday shoes. Different brands can come in slightly different lengths and, very importantly, widths.

Choose a cross-trainer, as these will be designed specifically for doing different types of workout (such as the ones in this book). Do not be swayed by fashion – no matter how good it looks, if it doesn't fit it will not do the job intended.

It is important to wear comfortable clothes that you can move freely in. Ideally, wear layers of breathable fabric, which can be taken off as your body temperature rises.

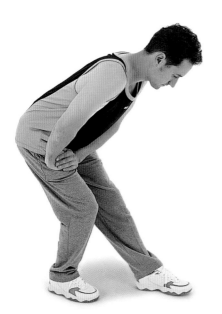

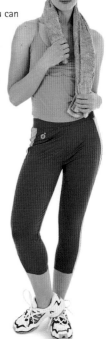

Warm-up Routine

It is vital to warm up before a workout, and to cool down and stretch afterwards (stretches before are optional). A basic warm-up should last at least 5 minutes. The rule is to start off slowly and build up. A warm-up helps to prevent injuries and it improves your performance.

It is also a time to prepare yourself for the workout to come, both physically and mentally. Use the time to focus on yourself. How does your body feel and how are you feeling at that moment? Are you feeling stiff? If so, spend longer on your warm-up. Any twinges? Be particularly careful about following the instructions.

Use the following exercises to help you warm up. Remember to start with minimal effort and build up gradually.

MARCHING ▽

1 Keep your feet softly flexed and don't 'slam' your feet down. Always keep your back straight and your abdominal muscles tight. Keeping your elbows bent, pump your arms keeping your fists soft.

2 Gradually quicken the pace and lift your knees slightly higher.

Repeat for 1 minute

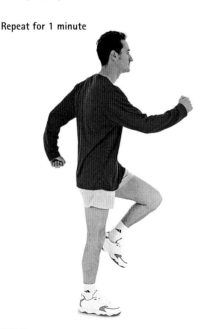

SHOULDER ROLLS ▽

While marching gently, roll your shoulders forward using their full range of motion. Let your arms hang at your sides and just let your shoulders do the work.

5 repetitions forwards then 5 backwards

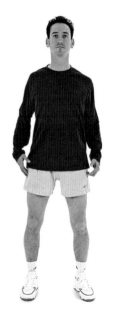

KNEE LIFTS ▷

Bring one knee at a time up to the opposite hand. Do not lean forwards or back. Keep your abdominal muscles tight and your back straight. Make sure your supporting knee is not locked out – keep it slightly soft.

Repeat for 1 minute

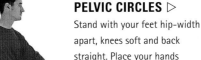

PELVIC CIRCLES ▷

Stand with your feet hip-width apart, knees soft and back straight. Place your hands above your hips and gently circle your pelvis in a 'D' shape – across the back and around the front. Try to isolate the movement to your hips only, keeping your knees and upper body as still as possible.

5 repetitions in each direction

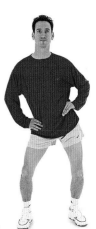

LEG CURLS ▽

1 Starting with legs wide apart, bring alternate heels towards your bottom. Make sure the knee of the supporting leg is soft and your footfall is gentle.

2 Begin punching both arms out in front of you in time with your leg movements.

Repeat for 1 minute

SQUATS ▽

1 Stand with your feet just over hip-width apart, knees soft and your bottom tucked under. Bend at the knees and hips and begin to squat down. Keep your back straight and your heels firmly on the ground. Make sure your knees travel in line with your toes and don't take your bottom any lower than the line of your knees.

2 Straighten up, making sure you do not lock out your knees at the top of the move.

Repeat for 1 minute

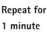

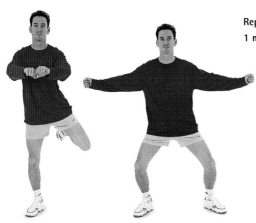

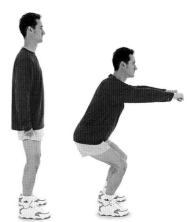

Cool-down Routine

Make sure you always finish a workout with a cool-down to allow the heart to recover at a safe pace. Top athletes never stand still after finishing an event, but always take time to walk around – this is called active recovery.

Do the following exercises for a minimum of 5 minutes to allow your heart rate and breathing to return to normal. Cooling down is also a great way to relax and focus on what you have achieved and how good you feel.

HALF STARS ▷

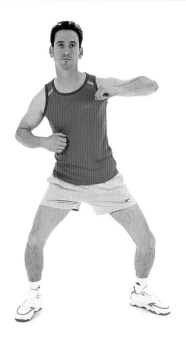

1 Start with your feet together and arms by your sides. Take your left leg out to the side, putting the foot flat on the floor and keeping the knee soft. At the same time lift the left arm out to the side in line with your shoulders.

2 Bring them both back to the centre and repeat with the right leg and right arm.

Repeat, alternating sides, for 1 minute

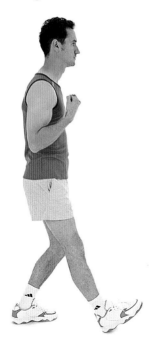

HEEL DIGS WITH BICEP CURLS ◁

Flex one foot and place the heel in front of you, keeping the supporting knee soft at all times. Alternate your feet and, as you dig each heel, curl both arms up to shoulder-height, keeping the elbows tucked neatly into your sides. Keep your back straight and your abdominals tight throughout.

Repeat for 1 minute

SIDE STEPS ▷

Start with your feet together and take two large steps out to your right. Immediately repeat back to the left. Keep your hands on your hips, back straight and abdominal muscles tight.

Repeat for 2 minutes

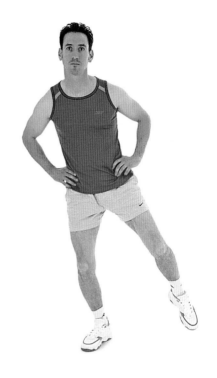

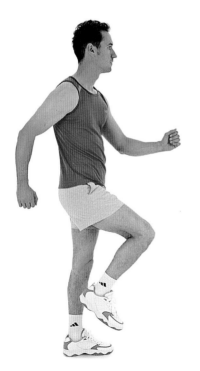

MARCHING ◁

March around, keeping your feet softly flexed and don't slam your feet down. Always keep your back straight and your abdominal muscles tight. With elbows bent, pump your arms softly. Take the tempo down slowly, at the same time decreasing arm and leg movements slowly.

Repeat for 1 minute

Stretches

Stretching is an important part of the cooling-down process of every workout as this is the most suitable time to stretch your muscles and gain optimum benefit. In the 30-Day Stomach-Toning Programme, stretches are included at the end of every workout. All stretching programmes (correctly done) aim to increase the mobility and elasticity of your muscles and thus prevent injuries occurring. Following a consistent stretching programme helps promote long, flexible muscles and, what's more, it will give you an all-over feeling of relaxed well-being.

End every workout by taking the time to stretch out every major muscle group. Your stretches are divided into two separate sections, one for the aerobic workouts and the other for the abdominal routines.

AEROBIC STRETCH ROUTINE

SEATED HAMSTRING STRETCH ▽

Sit on the floor with your left leg outstretched and the other tucked comfortably in. Make sure your hips are square on to the outstretched leg. Straighten your back, lifting your upper body and then take a deep breath in. As you breathe out stretch out over the straightened leg, placing your hands on your thighs with your arms bent. Keep the left foot gently flexed and try to keep the stretching leg as straight as possible – try not to let the back of the knee lift off the ground.

Hold for 15–20 seconds and then repeat with the other leg

TIPS FOR STRETCHING

• Hold each stretch for a minimum of 15 seconds.
• Stretch to a point of tension not pain.
• Keep breathing throughout.
• Movements must be performed slowly and under control.
• Keep warm by putting on extra layers of clothing if necessary.

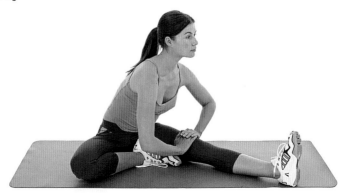

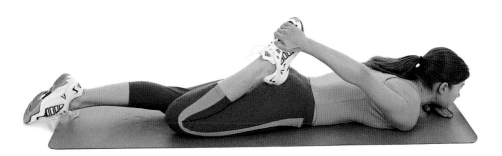

LYING QUAD STRETCH △

Lie on your front with your legs hip-width apart.
Place your left hand underneath your chin to act as a
cushion. Reach down with your right hand and gently
grasp your right foot drawing the heel towards the
buttock. Keep your knees and hips firmly on the
ground. You should feel the stretch along the
length of the front of your right thigh.

**Hold for 15–20 seconds and then repeat
on the other leg**

CALF STRETCH ◁

Stand with your feet hip-width
apart. Take one leg back, keeping
it straight, and bend the front knee
while pressing your front heel into
the ground. Keep your hips and
shoulders square and ensure your
feet stay hip-width apart. You
should feel this stretch in the
upper part of the back calf.

**Hold for 15–20 seconds and then
repeat with the other leg**

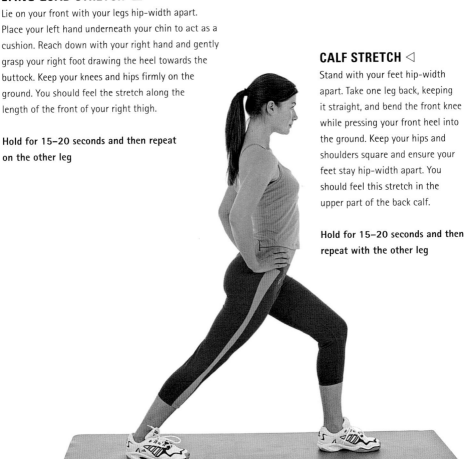

GLUT STRETCH ▽

1 Lie on your back with your back flat against the floor. Make sure your legs are hip-width apart, with your knees bent and the soles of your feet on the floor. Raise the right leg up and place it across the left leg. Your right shin should be resting on the fleshy upper part of the left knee.

2 Now bring the left leg upwards so that it is off the floor at almost 90 degrees. At the same time reach through and grasp your left thigh with both hands and gently draw the legs towards you.

Hold for 15–20 seconds and then repeat with the other leg

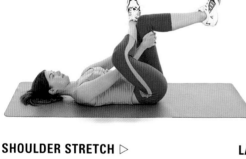

PECTORAL STRETCH ▽

Sit cross-legged on the floor. Place the palms of your hands on your lower back (fingers pointing downwards) and begin to squeeze your elbows together, letting your chest 'open'. Aim to feel the stretch across the front of the chest and the front of your shoulders.

Hold for 15 seconds

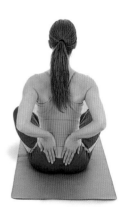

SHOULDER STRETCH ▷

Sit cross-legged on the floor. Swing your left arm across the front of your body and hook it in with your right forearm. Now gently draw the left arm across to feel a stretch in the back of the left shoulder.

Hold for 15 seconds and then repeat on the opposite side

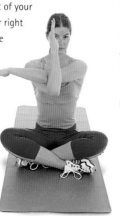

LAT STRETCH ▷

Sit cross-legged on the floor. Stretch both arms above your head and interlink your fingers. Stretch up through your arms feeling your ribcage lift slightly.

Hold for 15–20 seconds

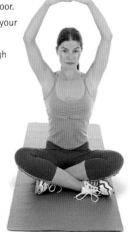

ABDOMINAL RESISTANCE STRETCH ROUTINE

SEATED WAIST ▷

Sit on the floor with your legs crossed. Place your left hand on the floor for support and then stretch your right hand up above your head. Straighten your back lifting your ribcage up and out of your hips, and now lean over to the left feeling a stretch along the right side of your body.

Hold for 15 seconds and then repeat on the other side

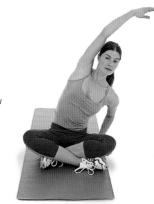

COBRA ▷

Lie on the floor on your front and place your hands flat on the floor with your thumbs level with your armpits. While breathing out, raise your head up slowly, arching your back. Try to keep the lower body motionless, heavy and strong. Feel your chest opening and your spine lengthening. Keep the movements slow.

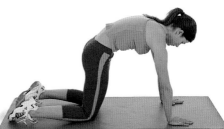

Hold for 10 seconds, return slowly to the floor and repeat

CAT CURLS ▽

1 Kneel with your hands on the floor, fingers pointing forwards and your hands directly under the line of your shoulders; your knees should be in line with your hips. Hollow your back, at the same time gently raising your head.

2 Slowly arch your back, vertebra by vertebra, into a hunch while dropping your head.

10 slow repetitions

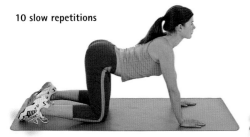

RESISTANCE WORKOUT

Getting started is always the biggest hurdle. Your next 30 days are carefully planned to ensure you get the best, and fastest, results possible. You will find that every day, even a rest day, contributes to your gaining optimum benefits. By alternating resistance workouts with aerobic workouts, you will be continually burning fat and improving your muscle tone. Although the build-up of workload is significant and will push you to achieve your best, you will find the next 30 days become a natural progression towards the end result – firm abs and a flat stomach!

Your first day begins with the basics. Don't be put off by these simple exercises; they are your foundation stones for all the work to come. Though they might look very simple, when performed correctly they are highly effective. Spend time getting comfortable with how your body feels when doing both exercises; remember slow and controlled are your key words.

AB TILTS ▷

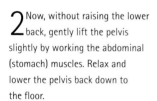

1 Lie on your back on the floor with your knees bent, arms resting at your sides and your feet flat on the floor. Your feet should be relatively close to your bottom so you are resting on your tailbone in a neutral spine position. Spend a few seconds becoming aware of how your spine feels resting on the floor.

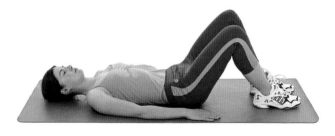

2 Now, without raising the lower back, gently lift the pelvis slightly by working the abdominal (stomach) muscles. Relax and lower the pelvis back down to the floor.

Level 1: 1 x 10 reps
Level 2: 2 x 10 reps

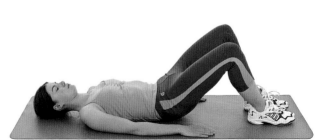

To cool down (see pages 40–41)   To stretch (see pages 42–45)

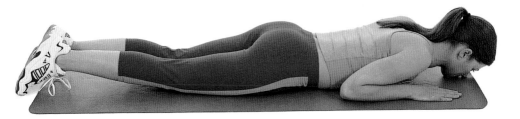

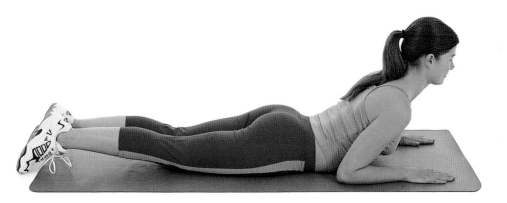

BACK EXTENSIONS △

1 Lie on your front and place your hands palms down by your shoulders. Your fingers are pointing forwards and elbows are on the ground.

2 Keeping your bottom and thighs relaxed, and chest pointing down towards the ground at all times, lift up pushing gently through your forearms. Return to the ground and repeat.

Level 1: 2 x 10 reps
Level 2: 2 x 15 reps

WHICH FITNESS LEVEL?

If you scored 5 or below in our fitness test (see pages 20–21), follow Level 1 in the resistance section. If you scored 6 or above, follow Level 2.

DAY 1 WORKOUT

	Level 1	Level 2
Ab Tilts	1 x 10 reps	2 x 10 reps
Back Extensions	2 x 10 reps	2 x 15 reps

Day 2

DON'T FORGET   To warm up (see pages 38–39)

FAST-PACED WALK 1

Here is where you get started on one of the three really important parts of your bid to obtain a beautiful body – the aerobic component. (The other two parts are the resistance workouts and improving your diet.) Today's activity is a fast-paced walk at 70 per cent MHR (see page 35), lasting for 25 minutes. Fast walking is a great way of keeping fit and burning off calories. It costs nothing and can often be fitted in more easily than other exercise routines.

Bear in mind that there are many ways to walk and that different speeds of walking burn different levels of calories – a gentle stroll will not make a marked difference. Walking a gentle 5 kph (3 mph) burns 70 calories in 20 minutes, but 7 kph (4.5 mph) for the same 20 minutes burns 90 calories, almost a 30 per cent increase. This is why it is important to keep the speed of your walking up. However, at the right pace, 1.5 km (1 mile) of walking can burn the same amount of calories as the same distance of jogging, even though it may take longer.

Follow these guidelines to make sure you get the most out of every walking workout.

Where to Walk

The simplest option is to step outside your front door and just get going, although it is a good idea to pre-plan your route. Where possible, choose somewhere you can walk without too much to distract you or to get in your way. A simple tip is to walk for 12–13 minutes in one direction and then turn around.

If you are lucky enough to be surrounded by green spaces or designated walking trails, then make the most of them. If you are going to go cross-country, then it is best to invest in a decent pair of walking boots. Trainers are not designed for the rigours of rocky terrain and mud. If you are town-based, then search out nearby open spaces and parks.

You can walk anywhere and get a great workout. You might even discover new places and sights that you would otherwise never have been aware of.

Good Walking Posture

Head and neck: keep your head centred between your shoulders, with your neck relaxed.

Shoulders and chest: your shoulders should be down and relaxed. Your chest and ribcage should be 'lifted'.

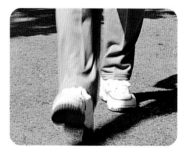

Arms and hands: bend your elbows to 90 degrees. Cup your hands gently, keeping them relaxed. Drive your elbows back as you walk, letting them skim the body. To go faster, pump your arms a bit quicker and your legs will follow.

Abdominals and lower back: pull your tummy muscles in but don't hold your breath.

Legs and feet: power the leg movements from your hips. Keep your knees soft and relax your ankles. Put your heel down and roll through: heel, ball then toe.

To cool down (see pages 40–41)   To stretch (see pages 42–45)

HIP ROLL TECHNIQUE

Practise the following technique as you are walking. You should feel your hip bones moving in a subtle, horizontal figure-of-eight pattern.

1 As you step out on your right heel, push your right hip forward.
2 After your right heel touches the ground, let the right hip pull the body forward.
3 As your right leg passes under you in mid-step, drop the right hip slightly. You should simultaneously drive the left hip forward.

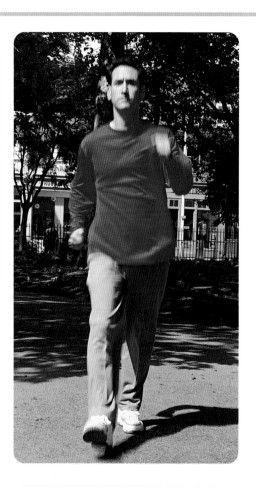

Advice on Technique

Don't overstride. Keep your stride a natural length and practise the hip roll technique (see above).
Keep knees straight but not locked out (hyperextended) for the duration of your walk.
Breathe deeply from your abdomen if you can.
Wear good shoes that support and cushion your feet well.
Wear comfortable clothes that can 'breathe' – natural fabrics where possible. Layers of clothes are ideal as they allow you to peel off items of clothing as you warm up.
Consider safety factors if you are going to walk in the dark. Be sensible and stick to well-lit and populated areas.
Do not listen to a personal stereo as you need to be aware of what is going on around you, whether it be traffic, cyclists or other people.

TECHNIQUE POINTS

• To step forward, plant your front heel on the ground, then roll your bodyweight through. Only when you have transferred your weight should the back leg begin to push.

• The buttocks get a great workout from fast-paced walking as they push you forwards. Try to think about using them to power you forwards.

RESISTANCE WORKOUT

Today we move on from the Ab Tilt exercise (see page 46), which showed how to engage the abdominal muscles, to learn how to do a Basic Sit-up, which actually works these muscles. It is important to remember what you learnt on Day 1 as the original exercises are a forerunner to the more advanced work to come.

You will need hand weights (see page 34) for the Side Bend exercises. These work the internal oblique muscles, helping you to bend to the side.

SIDE BENDS 1 ▽

1 Stand with your feet one-and-a-half times hip-width apart. Knees are soft, buttocks tucked under and your back is straight. Keep your shoulders relaxed and down.

2 Holding your hand weights in each hand, slowly stretch down to the right, taking care not to lean forwards or back. Aim to feel a stretch through the left side of your waist. Come slowly back up to the centre and repeat to the left. Keep the lower half of your body completely still at all times, with your weight evenly through both feet. Make sure the move is smooth and continuous.

Level 1: 1 x 20 reps each side
Level 2: 2 x 20 reps each side

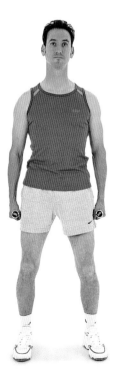
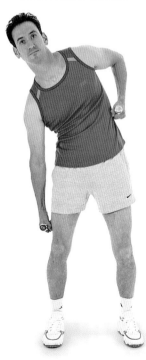

To cool down (see pages 40–41)   To stretch (see pages 42–45)

BASIC SIT-UPS ▷

1 Lie on the floor on your back, with your knees bent and your feet flat on the floor. Keep your feet relatively close to your bottom so that you are resting firmly on your tailbone with your spine in a neutral position. Keep your feet and knees hip-width apart. Place your hands at the base of your thighs, with palms facing down.

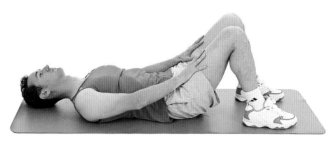

2 Lift your body up using your abdominals so that you lift your head, shoulders and then shoulder blades off the floor. Curl up slowly, running your hands up the length of your thighs. Breathe out as you do so to help the muscle contraction. Lower yourself slowly back down and breathe in.

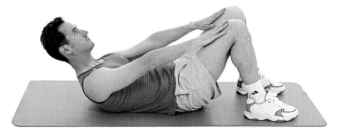

Level 1: 1 x 10 reps
Level 2: 2 x 10 reps

TECHNIQUE POINT

• Always try to visualize exactly what muscle you are working during your exercises. For example, when you are doing your Basic Sit-ups, think about pulling your stomach muscles tight and flat as well as how great they are going to look. During the Side Bends, consider how this exercise is going to improve your waist – it really works.

DAY 3 WORKOUT

	Level 1	Level 2
Side Bends 1	1 x 20 reps each side	2 x 20 reps each side
Ab Tilts (see page 46)	1 x 10 reps	2 x 10 reps
Back Extensions (see page 47)	2 x 10 reps	2 x 15 reps
Basic Sit-ups	1 x 10 reps	2 x 10 reps

EXERCISE TO MUSIC

Exercising to music is a popular and effective way to get fit. The following routine will push your heart rate up, make you hot and slightly sweaty (a good sign that you are working at the right level), and burn off calories. Aim to be working at 70 per cent MHR (see page 35).

STAR JUMPS ▷

1 Start with your feet hip-width apart and your arms by your sides.

2 Slightly bend the knees and jump out landing with your feet one-and-half times hip-width apart. Make sure you land with slightly bent knees, sinking into the move to absorb excess impact. At the same time lift your arms up and above your head, keeping a slight bend in your elbows. Immediately jump back to the start position and repeat.

Repeat for 2 minutes

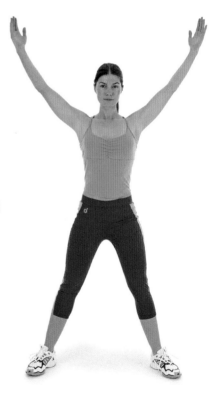

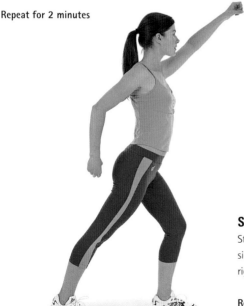

SPOTTY DOGS ◁

Start with your feet hip-width apart, arms by your sides. Jump, throwing both your right leg and your right arm forwards and then swap to the other side.

Repeat for 2 minutes

SIDE LUNGES ▷

1 Start with your feet hip-width apart, and your arms by your sides. Now lunge to the right with the right foot turning the body slightly towards the left. At the same time stretch the right arm out and across the body. The left arm swings naturally back behind the body.

2 Return immediately to the start position and do the same to the other side.

Repeat for 2 minutes

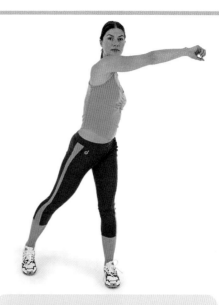

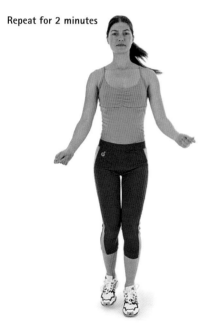

VIRTUAL SKIPPING △

Pretend you have a skipping rope and skip from foot to foot. If you want to work the upper body, then do the arm movements too.

Repeat for 2 minutes

TECHNIQUE POINTS

• Make sure you maintain good posture during the entire workout. Think of keeping your back straight and abdominal muscles tight throughout.

• Move about the room as much as possible. Impact is lessened on the body's joints if you don't stay on one spot.

DAY 4 WORKOUT

Do this routine 3 times so you have completed a total of 24 minutes plus your warm-up and cool-down exercises and stretches.

ALTERNATIVE WORKOUT

Fast-paced walk for 25 minutes at 70 per cent MHR (see page 35).

RESISTANCE WORKOUT

Good strong tummy muscles are achieved through a variety of exercises. Engaging your abdominals is just part of the work; it is also important to make sure the opposite muscle group – the lower back – is strong and toned. Today's workout includes an exercise to strengthen the lower back in the shape of the Superman exercise – don't giggle, it really works.

SIDE CURLS ▷

1 Lie on the floor flat on your back and bend your knees. Place your feet relatively close to your bottom so that you are resting firmly on your tailbone in a neutral spine position.

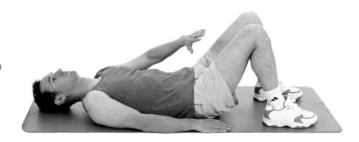

2 Curl up slowly, holding your stomach in and twisting your torso to reach your left arm across the body, towards your right knee. Breathe out as you come up and hold your stomach in. Lower your body under control and repeat immediately. Work one side at a time, moving the same hand towards the opposite knee. Remember to keep your chin off your chest at all times.

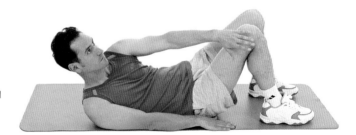

Level 1: 1 x 10 reps each side
Level 2: 2 x 10 reps each side

SUPERMAN 1 ▽

1 Lie on the floor on your front with your arms outstretched in front of you. Keep your nose pointing down to the ground.

2 Lift your left arm and right leg simultaneously off the floor. Resist the urge to throw them up; this isn't a big move so try to keep it slow and controlled at all times. Return them to the ground and immediately repeat using the right arm and left leg.

Level 1: 1 x 10 reps
Level 2: 2 x 10 reps

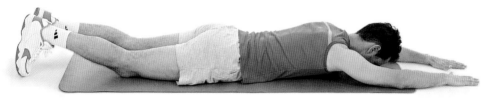

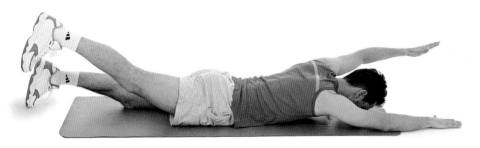

DAY 5 WORKOUT

	Level 1	Level 2
Side Bends 1 (see page 50)	1 x 20 reps each side	2 x 20 reps each side
Basic Sit-ups (see page 51)	1 x 10 reps	2 x 10 reps
Back Extensions (see page 47)	2 x 10 reps	2 x 15 reps
Side Curls	1 x 10 reps each side	2 x 10 reps each side
Superman 1	1 x 10 reps	2 x 10 reps

TECHNIQUE POINT

• Try to visualize strengthening your lower back muscles during the Superman exercise. Similarly, during the Side Curls, picture toning your obliques, the muscles at the side of your stomach.

STEP AEROBIC ROUTINE

This is the last exercise day before you get a well-deserved rest day, so try to make an extra effort. Any form of step aerobics adds variation to your workout and you will be surprised how it can increase the intensity of your exercise routine.

Do these exercises to music, but be aware that some music will be too fast, so regulate the pace if necessary. Step aerobic videos are also a good way to keep boredom at bay. Make sure you have enough room – at least two square metres.

BASIC STEP ▷

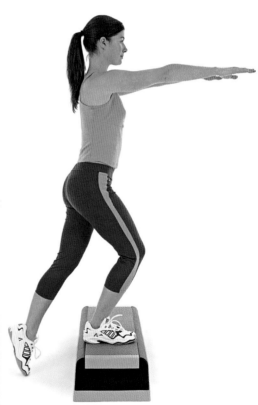

1 Step up and down on to your step. Lead with one foot for 10 steps to begin with and then change over. Continue this simple combination for the whole 5 minutes. Make sure you put your whole foot on the step (don't let your heel drop off the edge) and keep your knees slightly bent. Also, think about your posture throughout – stand tall, with shoulders back, and use your arms to pump you forwards and up.

2 To make the workout harder add arm movements. Pump them straight out in front or (even harder) pump them above the head. Remember to keep a slight bend in your elbows.

Repeat for 5 minutes

TECHNIQUE POINT

• Always wear trainers when doing step aerobics and have water to hand so you can keep yourself hydrated throughout.

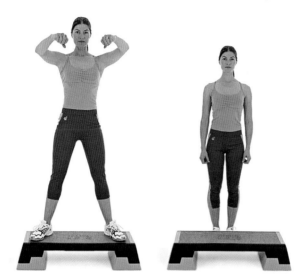

V-STEP ◁

1 Step up on to your step leading with the right foot. Take the foot wide as if to create part of a V-shape. Follow up immediately with the left foot to create the other side of the V.

2 Step back down (right foot, left foot) to a normal hip-width apart stance and repeat with the same leg leading. Do 10 V-steps, leading with the right leg. March on the spot for a few seconds and then change to lead with the left foot.

Repeat for 5 minutes

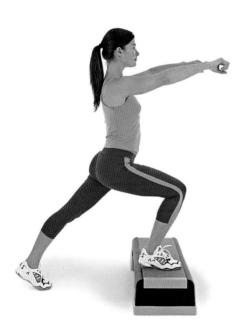

LUNGES ◁

Start by standing on the step, facing forwards. Lunge off backwards, first to the left letting the toe tap down on the floor before stepping back up. Quickly follow with the other foot. Let your arms swing naturally across the body during this movement.
Keep your abdominal muscles tight and your back straight throughout.

Repeat for 3 minutes

DAY 6 WORKOUT

Do this routine twice so you have completed 26 minutes plus your warm-up and cool-down exercises and stretches.

ALTERNATIVE WORKOUT

A 30-minute fast-paced walk at 70 per cent MHR (see page 35).

REST DAY

Well done! You have reached your first day of rest with no workouts to perform. However, if you do feel like going for a gentle walk or swim with the kids there is no reason why you shouldn't. Give yourself a mental pat on the back for completing your first week so successfully and reward yourself for a job well done. Resist the temptation to gorge yourself on your favourite food – instead treat yourself to a massage, a wander around the shops or try the simple breathing exercise below as part of an enjoyable relaxation session.

Because of the calming effect of any breathing exercise, you can use them any time or place. So next time you are feeling stressed or just overwhelmed, hide yourself away for a few minutes and do some deep breathing.

THE WHISPERED 'AH' ▷

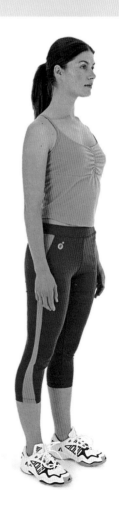

1 This Alexander Technique exercise is a great way of becoming aware of your breath. It can be done either standing or sitting, but is best done standing. Find a warm, quiet room and make sure you won't be disturbed. Stand in the middle of the room, facing a window if possible. Looking at a view will help you to relax. To start, mentally scan your body, running through the following checklist:

• Spread your weight evenly over both feet and relax your ankles.

• Relax your knees and make sure they are not locked.

• Relax your hips and let your pelvis drop freely towards the floor.

• Relax your tummy muscles.

• Drop your shoulders and hang your arms freely by your sides.

• Relax your neck.

2 Once you have gone over this mental checklist, let your jaw drop open, with your tongue resting lightly behind your lower teeth. Think of something nice and smile a little. Now, breathe out gently on a whispered 'Ah', until you have run out of breath. There should be very little sound. If you hear any vocalized sound you are probably holding on to some tension.

3 Close your mouth and instead of immediately breathing in, think of doing nothing, and you will find your ribs spring out of their own accord. Do not be surprised if you feel a little dizzy. If you do, stop for a moment before continuing.

Repeat the whole process 5 times

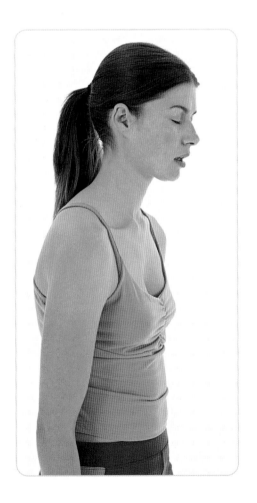

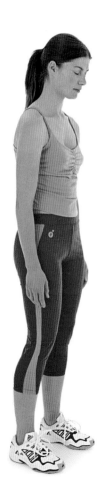

RESISTANCE WORKOUT

Your rest day should have left you feeling refreshed and raring to go. This is a good time to go over your motivational lists (see pages 18–19) and re-read last week's food diary (see page 29). Try to spot any weak points you have during the day – maybe a mid-afternoon sugar craving or a nightly glass of wine. Whatever it is, try to find your own solution. A bit of lateral thinking should yield some inventive yet effective ideas to help you on your way.

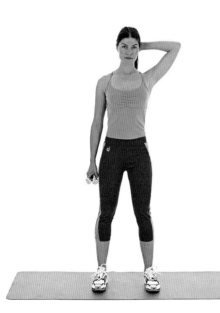 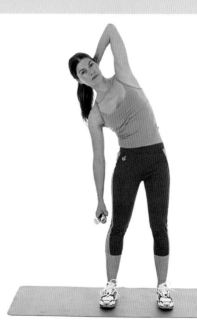

SIDE BENDS 2 △

1 Stand with your feet one-and-half times hip-width apart. Your knees are soft, buttocks tucked under and your back is straight. Keep your shoulders relaxed and down. Hold a set of hand weights (see page 34) in your right hand and place your left hand up by your left ear.

2 Now stretch down to the right taking care not to lean forwards or back. Feel a stretch along the left side of your body. Come slowly back up to the start position and repeat on the same side. Keep the lower half of your body completely still at all times, weight even through both feet. Keep the move slow and continuous. When you have completed the required repetitions, change sides.

Level 1: 1 x 15 reps each side
Level 2: 2 x 15 reps each side

SIT-UPS ▷

1 Lie flat on your back on the floor with knees bent and your feet flat on the floor. Keep your feet relatively close to your bottom so that you are resting firmly on your tailbone with your spine in a neutral position. Keep your feet and knees hip-width apart. Cup your hands by your ears letting your elbows fall out.

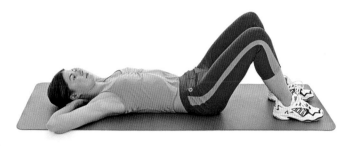

2 Now, lift your body up from your abdominals – lift your head, shoulders and then shoulder blades off the floor. Curl up slowly, keeping your chin off your chest. Breathe out as you lift up. Lower yourself slowly back down and inhale.

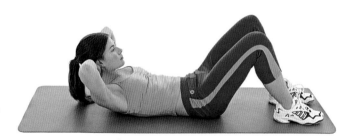

Level 1: 2 x 10 reps
Level 2: 2 x 15 reps

DAY 8 WORKOUT

	Level 1	Level 2
Side Bends 2	1 x 15 reps each side	2 x 15 reps each side
Sit-ups	2 x 10 reps	2 x 15 reps
Back Extensions (see page 47)	2 x 10 reps	2 x 15 reps
Side Curls (see page 54)	1 x 10 reps each side	2 x 10 reps each side
Superman 1 (see page 55)	1 x 10 reps	2 x 10 reps

TECHNIQUE POINT

• If you have a full-length mirror to hand, use it to check your posture and technique as you exercise.

INTERVAL TRAINING

Interval training involves periods of high-intensity effort followed by recovery periods of less intense activity. It has been a successful training trick of both professional and amateur athletes for years and, no matter how fit you are, it is a good way to improve cardiovascular fitness and lose body fat. It is great way to kick-start your metabolism and burn a lot of calories.

There are two levels of interval training: firstly anaerobic (without oxygen) and secondly aerobic (with oxygen). Anaerobic interval training involves working a muscle to complete failure or fatigue, as in sprinting or strenuous weight training, and is for people who are extremely fit.

Aerobic interval training involves working the muscles but not to fatigue. This is what you are going to do today with a 30-minute running and walking workout. This involves running for 1 minute, then recovering using a 2-minute walk and repeating the process 10 times.

THE WORKOUT

1 Make sure you warm up either by following the warm-up routine or by working up from a gentle stroll to a brisk walk over 5 minutes. Either use a stopwatch or just keep a careful eye on your watch.

2 Walk briskly for 2 minutes.

3 Break into a gentle run for 1 minute. After the minute is up, slow back down into your fast walk, but make sure it is as brisk a walk as you started with.

4 Repeat the whole process 10 times in all so you achieve a 30-minute workout in addition to your initial warm-up.

5 Make sure you spend another 5 minutes cooling down and letting your heart rate return to normal. If at any point during the workout you feel out of breath or dizzy return to a fast walk until you are suitably recovered.

Wear good trainers to cushion and support your feet and ankles. Don't try too hard – it may be very tempting to go charging off during your first running phase but you will probably end up out of breath and will definitely put more strain on your joints.

Benefits of Interval Training

• You will burn more calories. Interval training uses mainly carbohydrates rather than fat for energy, but because of its increased intensity level it still burns more calories overall.

• You will be able to achieve more in each workout. Interval training increases the amount of high-intensity work you can do each time, as you get a chance to recover between sessions.

• You will improve your cardiovascular fitness and your body's ability to manage lactic acid.

To cool down (see pages 40–41)   To stretch (see pages 42–45)

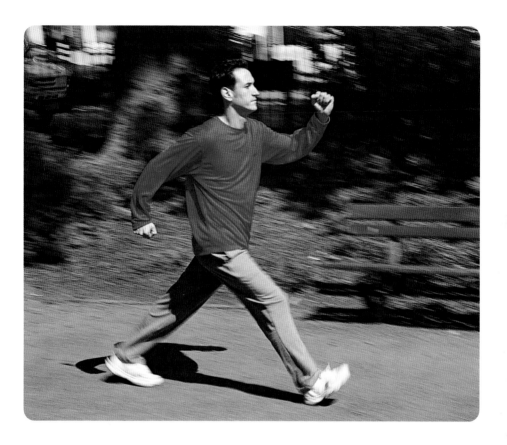

TECHNIQUE POINTS

• Short fast strides are better than long ones.

• Keep your feet close to the ground.

• Land on your heels, then roll through your foot.

• Keep the body upright and straight, tummy muscles pulled in.

DAY 9 WORKOUT

Alternate 2 minutes of brisk walking with 1 minute of gentle running 10 times so the workout lasts for 30 minutes. Don't forget to warm up and cool down properly as well.

Day 10

DON'T FORGET To warm up (see pages 38–39)

RESISTANCE WORKOUT

Today's new exercise – the Sit-up and Twist – begins to target your external oblique muscle (see page 15). The primary function of this muscle is to bend the spine to the same side and to rotate the torso to the opposite side. While you are doing the Sit-up and Twist, visualize yourself whittling away at the waist and you will help improve your technique and see faster results. The Back Extension is a more advanced version of the one from Day 1 (see page 47). With no help from the forearms, the lower back has to do all the work this time.

SIT-UP AND TWIST ▷

1 Lie on the floor on your back, with your knees up. Press your lower back into the floor, if necessary, so that your spine is in a neutral position. Cup your ears with your hands. Place your right ankle over your left upper knee.

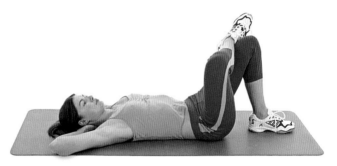

2 Keeping your lower body as still as possible, take your left shoulder towards the right knee. Keep your chin off your chest and breathe out as you lift up. Hold for a split second at the top of the move (make sure both hips remain firmly on the ground) and then return slowly to the start position. Repeat immediately.

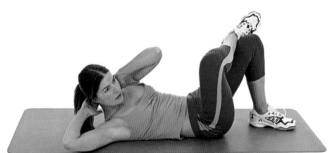

Level 1: 1 x 10 reps each side
Level 2: 1 x 20 reps each side

To cool down (see pages 40–41)   To stretch (see pages 42–45)

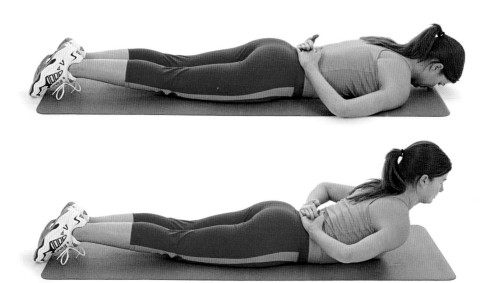

BACK EXTENSIONS (NO ARMS) △

1 Lie on your front and place your hands in the small of your back.

Level 1: 2 x 10 reps
Level 2: 2 x 15 reps

2 Keeping your bottom and thighs relaxed, and chest pointing down towards the ground at all times, lift your chest off the ground. Return slowly to the floor and repeat immediately.

TECHNIQUE POINT

• This is a small movement and to begin with you may only be able to lift a couple of centimetres (an inch or so) – this is perfectly normal. As your back strengthens you will find it easier to lift higher. Keep the move slow and controlled and don't force it. Concentrate on keeping your bottom and legs relaxed. Let your lower back do the work.

DAY 10 WORKOUT

	Level 1	Level 2
Side Bends 2 (see page 60)	1 x 15 reps each side	2 x 15 reps each side
Sit-ups (see page 61)	2 x 10 reps	2 x 15 reps
Back Extensions (no arms)	2 x 10 reps	2 x 15 reps
Sit-up and Twist	1 x 10 reps each side	1 x 20 reps each side
Superman 1 (see page 55)	1 x 10 reps	2 x 10 reps

REBOUNDER WORKOUT

Using a rebounder is great aerobic exercise especially for anyone with joint problems as it doesn't jar the ankles, knees and lower back in the same way that hitting solid ground does. It also burns calories, tones your body, improves your balance and increases your agility.

Try to jump from and land on the middle of the rebounder. Any jumping exercise can wreak havoc with a weak pelvic floor so build up gradually if you have ever had problems with your bladder or stress incontinence. Set an alarm or timer, put on some music and off you go!

WALKING

Start by simply walking your feet through to get used to how it feels – press your heels deep into the rebounder.

Repeat for 2 minutes

JOGGING ▷

Begin to build up the intensity by jogging slowly. Keep your arms quite close to your body but still moving freely. When you begin to feel more confident, start lifting your knees a bit higher and add a little jump as you land.

Repeat for 2 minutes

TWISTING ▽

Twist from side to side using your abdominals and tighten them with every twist. Keep your knees soft. Start using your arms by punching them out with every move you make.

Repeat for 2 minutes

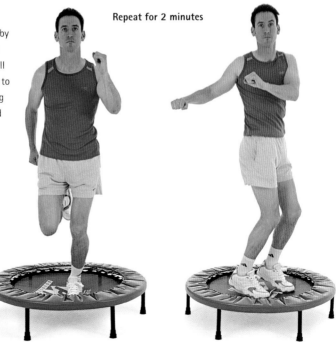

To cool down (see pages 40–41)   To stretch (see pages 42–45)

KNEE LIFTS ▷

Bring your opposite hand towards your opposite knee. Keep your back straight and your abdominals tight at all times. To make it harder, add a small hop with every knee lift.

Repeat for 2 minutes

TUCK JUMPS ▷

This one is more difficult than it sounds, so be careful. As you jump up, try to draw your knees to your chest. Keep your back as straight as possible and pull your abdominals tight.

Repeat for 2 minutes

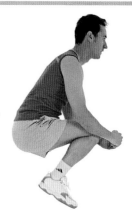

STAR JUMPS ▷

Take off with both feet and, as you lift upwards spread both your arms and legs out to the side in a star position.

Repeat for 2 minutes

TECHNIQUE POINTS

• Keep your knees slightly bent throughout.

• To avoid aching calves, press your heels all the way down as you land.

DAY 11 WORKOUT

Warm up before you start then do the routine twice, trying to keep going for at least 25 minutes.

ALTERNATIVE WORKOUT

Do a fast-paced walk or gentle jog for 30 minutes at 80 per cent MHR (see page 35).

DON'T FORGET   To warm up (see pages 38–39)

RESISTANCE WORKOUT

There are just two more days before your next well-earned rest day. You might be needing it, but don't despair – feeling slightly stiff is perfectly normal and it shows just how hard you have been working. With regular exercise, it will happen less and less often. Don't be tempted to over-do it though – there is a major difference between feeling stiff and being in pain.

Delayed Onset Muscle Soreness (DOMS) is a term coined to explain the stiffness you may feel 24–48 hours after exercising. This can vary from not being able to walk downstairs properly to acute pain. If you find yourself suffering from the latter, then ease off for a couple of days. Halve the sets and repetitions until you return to normal and never exercise if you feel in pain.

THREE-QUARTER PLANK ▷

1 Begin on your hands and knees, with your hands under your shoulders and your knees under your hips.

2 Walk back on your knees until you are resting on the fleshy part just above your kneecaps. Your back should be straight and your abdominal muscles tight. Keep your shoulders back and down and your arms straight. Do not lock your elbows. Hold.

Level 1: 1 x 5 breaths
Level 2: 2 x 5 breaths

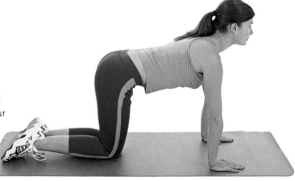

TECHNIQUE POINT

• Instead of sets and repetitions, you can either count your breaths (1 in and out counts as 1 breath) or just count slowly to the required number.

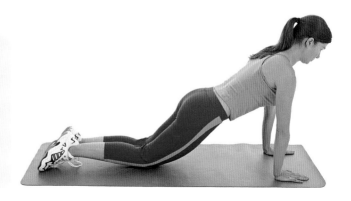

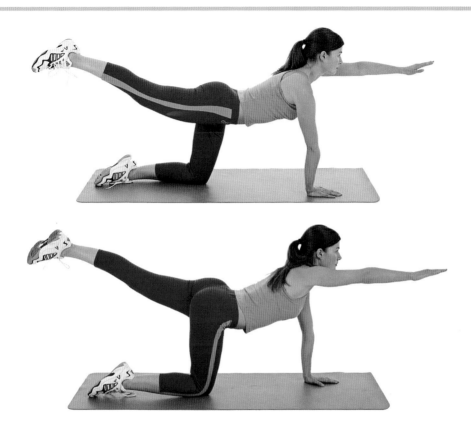

SUPERMAN 2 △

1 Start off on your hands and knees. Position your hands under your shoulders and knees under your hips. Tighten your abdominals and keep your back as straight as possible throughout.

2 Lift your left arm and your right leg up in a straight line, then return to the start position and repeat with the right arm and the left leg.

Level 1: 2 x 10 reps
Level 2: 2 x 16 reps

DAY 12 WORKOUT

	Level 1	Level 2
Side Bends 1 (see page 50)	1 x 20 reps each side	2 x 20 reps each side
Sit-ups (see page 61)	2 x 10 reps	2 x 15 reps
Back Extensions (no arms – see page 65)	2 x 10 reps	2 x 15 reps
¾ Plank	1 x 5 breaths	2 x 5 breaths
Superman 2	2 x 10 reps	2 x 16 reps
Sit-up and Twist (see page 64)	1 x 10 reps each side	1 x 20 reps each side

DON'T FORGET   To warm up (see pages 38–39)

SKIPPING

Skipping is an excellent way to keep fit, and can be done almost anywhere, anytime. It will improve your cardiovascular fitness, flexibility and co-ordination. It is great for the legs and buttocks, and for building bones.

It is important to make sure your rope is the correct length for your height. To check the length, stand on the middle of the rope and pull the handles upwards until the rope is taut. The handles should come to the middle of the chest. If they come above chest level, the rope will need shortening. Make sure your trainers provide adequate cushioning for the ball of your foot.

Practice and Warm-up

Even if you haven't skipped for a long time, spend 5 minutes easing yourself in before you get started properly. After your warm-up, start by jumping on the spot on the balls of your feet. Begin by practising your timing, then try this exercise: hold both handles of the rope in one hand and rotate it in a circular movement to your side. When the rope hits the ground, jump. Progress to jumping over the rope once you are confident your timing is correct.

Skipping is surprisingly strenuous, so start slowly. Practise by skipping for 20–30 seconds, then marching on the spot for 30 seconds and repeating. As your fitness improves you can increase the length of time you skip for. Make sure you master the basic jumps before moving on to more complicated ones.

Always remember to give your lower-leg muscles a really thorough stretch after skipping.

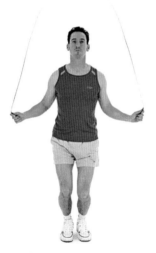

BASIC JUMP △

Stand upright and keep your abdominal muscles tight. Hold the rope with hands out to the side and elbows in. Swing the rope continuously over your head. As the rope comes towards the floor, push off from the balls of your feet and jump over it. Jump only about 2.5 cm (1 in) off the floor and keep your knees slightly bent.

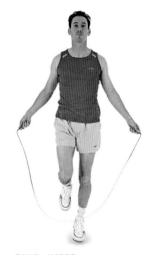

SKIP JUMP △

Hop on one foot per rope revolution while lifting (kicking) the other foot out in front (or behind) the body. Alternate legs with each revolution and stay close to the floor.

HOP JUMP ▽

Hop on one leg for several jumps, and then alternate legs (start with 2 hop jumps per leg and increase as you improve).

SKI JUMP ▷

Start with a basic jump. Keeping your feet together, jump left to right across an imaginary line (side to side). Keep your knees slightly bent and increase the width of your jumps as you improve.

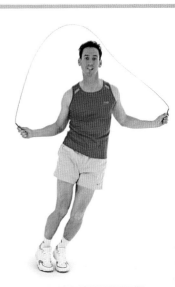

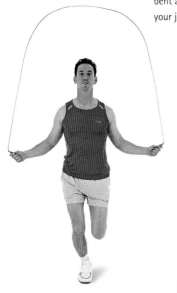

TECHNIQUE POINTS

• Never hunch over. Keep your back straight, abdominal muscles tight and your head up.

• Jump low, about 2.5 cm (1 in) off the ground, to minimize the impact on your knees and ankles.

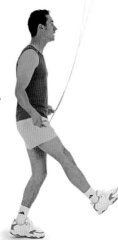

KICK JUMP ▷

Start with a basic jump, then kick your foot in front, alternating legs. Keep the kicking foot gently flexed.

DAY 13 WORKOUT

Aim to skip for at least 20 minutes but don't be put off by teething problems. It is normal to take a while even to get 10 or 20 skips in a row. If you find yourself becoming hopelessly out of breath, stop and march it through for a few minutes and then try again.

ALTERNATIVE WORKOUT

Do a fast walk or jog for 30 minutes at 80 per cent MHR (see page 35).

REST DAY

You are nearly half-way through the programme and you thoroughly deserve your rest day. Make it really special and mentally rewarding by actively concentrating on de-stressing and relaxing. Try not to spend the day running around catching up on too many chores, but if you have no choice make sure you set aside some time for yourself.

The ancient discipline of meditation involves contemplation while focusing your mind on a thought or object. It is a form of conscious and chosen relaxation which can help you understand everything in your life more clearly. If you have never tried meditating before, why don't you give it a go? It is much easier than you might think.

Create the Right Environment

This depends on your living space. Ideally, pick a quiet place in your home that you can return to again and again. This space should be pleasant, naturally lit, uncluttered and a comfortable temperature. Do your best to avoid distractions: take the phone off the hook or put a 'do not disturb' sign on the door.

Finding a Suitable Position

Becoming relaxed is the first part of preparing to meditate so make sure you are comfortable and not inclined to fidget. How you sit is up to you; try a hard-backed chair or cross-legged on a soft rug or cushion. Keep your back straight and shoulders pulled gently back. Either clasp your hands or just place them in your lap.

THE MEDITATION

1 Start breathing slowly and deeply. Now repeat the following words to yourself, and start to feel the tension release:

The muscles of my neck are relaxing; I am relaxed.
The muscles of my shoulders and chest are relaxing;
I am relaxed.
The muscles of my arms and hands are relaxing;
I am relaxed.
The muscles of my legs and feet are relaxing;
I am relaxed.
My mind is calm. My body is calm. I am relaxed.
My mind is alert. My mind is awake.

2 Once you are physically relaxed, you can begin to meditate inwardly. There are lots of ways to do this but the principle in general is to keep your mind focused on one subject, something which can be surprisingly hard. One technique that is worth trying is taking an 'inner' voyage similar to the one given here. Read it and then create your own version.

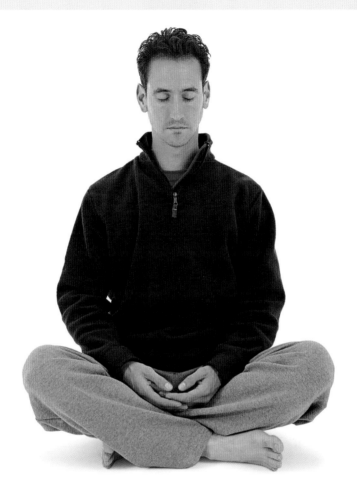

You are standing at a gate on a sunny summer's day. The gate leads into a large flower-covered field. You walk through the gate up to the large central tree that dominates the field. What does the tree look like? Touch the bark and then pick either a leaf or a flower. Finally, sit with your back up against the tree and meditate on the tree itself. Feel a soft warm wind on your face. To close, retrace your steps and allow the image to dissolve.

There are many other things you can visualize; some may be more appropriate for you personally. Choose a place that fills you with harmony and relaxation. Try to start with a 5-minute meditation and progress to longer sessions from there.

DON'T FORGET   To warm up (see pages 38–39)

RESISTANCE WORKOUT

The third week begins with a new move: Reverse Curls. These exercises will feel as though you are targeting the lower half of your abdominals (the ones below your navel).

The second exercise, Twisting Abs, is the next level up in terms of difficulty and control, as you have to stop mid-move for a split second, which will require the use of your new-found muscle strength. Remember to keep breathing all the way through and make sure you are completely focused on isolating your abdominal muscles (not your lower-back or thigh muscles).

REVERSE CURLS ▽

1 Lie on the floor on your back. Raise your legs in the air until they are straight but the knees are not locked out. Press your heels towards the ceiling, gently flexing the feet. Place your hands at your sides, palms facing up. Pull your stomach in tightly and press the spine into the floor.

2 Using your abdominal muscles, lift the hips off the ground and then lower them back down again. Remember to concentrate on lifting your pelvis up towards your stomach – not simply raising and lowering your legs. Keep the movement smooth and try not to rock your body.

Level 1: 1 x 20 reps
Level 2: 2 x 20 reps

TECHNIQUE POINT

• Make sure you are using only the strength in your abdomen to do this exercise. Even a very small move is effective.

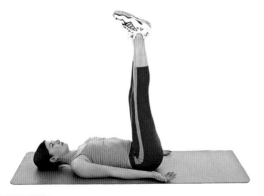
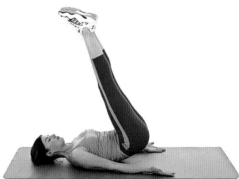

To cool down (see pages 40–41)   To stretch (see pages 42–45)

TWISTING ABS ▷

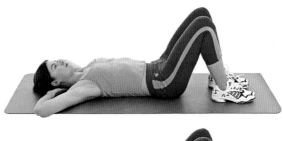

1 Lie on the floor with your back flat, knees bent and feet flat on the floor. Keep your feet relatively close to your bottom so that you are resting firmly on your tailbone with your spine in a neutral position. Keep your feet and knees hip-width apart. Cup your hands by your ears letting your elbows fall out naturally.

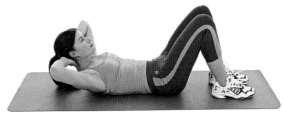

2 Now, lift your body up from your abdominals so that you lift your head, shoulders and then shoulder blades off the floor. Curl up slowly, breathing out as you do so. Hold at the top of the move for 1 second.

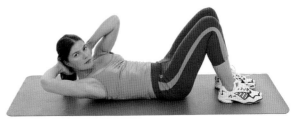

3 Then, twist your left shoulder towards your right knee, hold for 1 second and then return slowly to the centre. Turn the right shoulder to the left knee, then return to the centre and lower yourself to the starting position.

Level 1: 1 x 20 reps
Level 2: 2 x 20 reps

DAY 15 WORKOUT

	Level 1	Level 2
Side Bends 2 (see page 60)	1 x 15 reps each side	2 x 15 reps each side
Sit-ups (see page 61)	2 x 10 reps	2 x 15 reps
Back Extensions (no arms – see page 65)	2 x 10 reps	2 x 15 reps
¾ Plank (see page 68)	1 x 5 breaths	2 x 5 breaths
Sit-up and Twist (see page 64)	1 x 10 reps each side	1 x 20 reps each side
Superman 2 (see page 69)	2 x 10 reps	2 x 16 reps
Twisting Abs	1 x 20 reps	2 x 20 reps

DON'T FORGET   To warm up (see pages 38–39)

FAST-PACED WALK 2

Today's workout is a 40-minute fast-paced walk at 80 per cent MHR (see page 35). Ideally, pre-plan your route to include whatever constitutes 'countryside' in your local area. This might be anything from a local nature reserve to a large park. If you are lucky enough to live within striking distance of the countryside then this would make the best walk.

Why? Research and experience show that there are huge benefits to be gained from walking outdoors, and the greener your surroundings the better. It is a sensory experience to exercise out in the fresh air, and sunlight tops up Vitamin D levels, which are essential for bone growth and development among other things. Walking also helps to eliminate stress hormones called catecholamines (the best known of these is adrenaline) from the body. Finally, walking is low-impact so it puts little strain on the joints and is a great lower-body workout.

The Practicalities of Walking

Having obtained information about your area and possible walking trails, decide exactly where you want to walk. Always consider safety: tell a friend or relative your exact route in case of an emergency. Check the weather forecast before you head out and take some supplies with you; in particular a full water bottle and some plasters for emergency blister treatment are especially useful.

It is a good idea to wear clothes that can 'breathe' so choose natural fabrics and layer your clothes so you can peel off as you warm up. If you are walking long-distance or on uneven terrain, it is worth investing in a good pair of walking boots. It is important to ensure a good fit. Put your full weight on your feet while you are being fitted and wear walking socks while trying them on. Check your heel has minimal lift and that your toes do not rub against the front. Finally ensure the ankle is well padded and your foot feels secure. It is a good idea to wear your boots a little before you embark on a long walk.

When you are walking, be sure to look out for unexpected changes in terrain, such as tree roots that stick out and steep banks, to avoid stumbling or tripping over.

Making it Harder

There will come a point in your walking workout when you begin to find walking on the flat easier. Now is the time (if you would rather not jog or run) when it is important to 'up' the intensity. You can do this by adding incline – change your route to take in some gradual inclines or, later on, hills. You will be surprised how even the most subtle incline can make a big difference to your workout. Alternatively you could try hillwalking – find a steep hill and stride up it at a hard pace for 1–2 minutes, turn around and walk back down and repeat. Begin by doing this 3–4 times. Eventually you can increase the length of time of your climbing period to 3–4 minutes and so on.

TECHNIQUE POINTS

• Stand up straight with your torso aligned over your hips.

• As you walk, focus your eyes about 3.5 m (12 ft) in front of you.

To cool down (see pages 40—41)   To stretch (see pages 42—45)

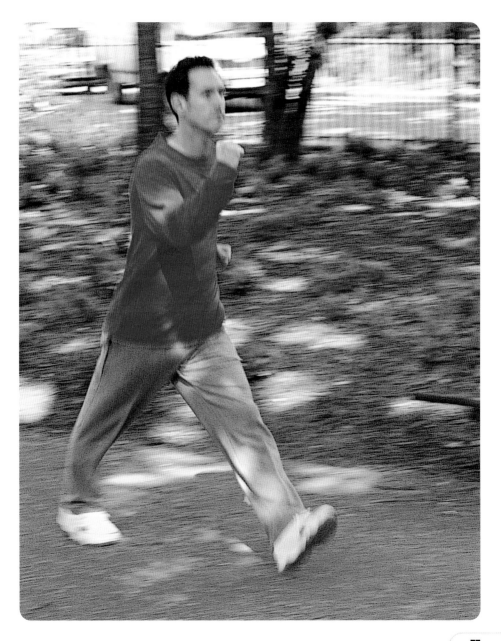

Day 17

DON'T FORGET   To warm up (see pages 38–39)

RESISTANCE WORKOUT

Today's new exercise looks deceptively easy, but don't be fooled. The Plank targets our core stability muscles (see page 14), which are some of the hardest-working muscles in the body. Although they are the primary source of balance, posture and overall body strength, as well as being essential to the body's movement and fluidity, they can be hard to isolate during a workout. There is also an advanced variation on the Sit-up and Twist exercise from Day 10 (see page 64).

THE PLANK ▽

Begin on your hands and knees. Position your hands under your shoulders, and your knees under your hips. Take your feet back until your legs are straight and you are balancing on your toes, with your feet together. Keep your shoulders back and down and your arms straight. Do not lock out your elbows. Hold.

Level 1: 1 x 10 breaths
Level 2: 2 x 10 breaths

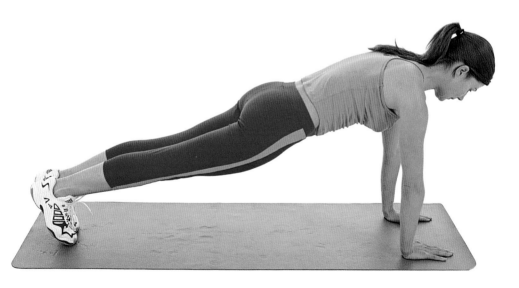

To cool down (see pages 40–41)   To stretch (see pages 42–45)

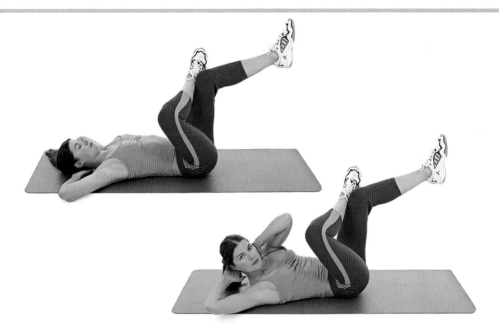

SIT-UP AND TWIST (FEET OFF FLOOR) △

1 Lie on your back on the floor, and press your lower back into the floor if necessary, making sure your spine is in a neutral position. Place both hands by your ears. Lift up your left leg to form a right angle with the floor and place your right ankle over your left upper knee.

2 While keeping your legs as still as possible, take your left shoulder towards your right knee. Keep your chin off your chest and breathe out as you lift up. Perform for the desired repetitions and then change to the other side.

Level 1: 1 x 20 reps each side
Level 2: 2 x 20 reps each side

DAY 17 WORKOUT

	Level 1	Level 2
Side Bends 1 (see page 50)	1 x 20 reps each side	2 x 20 reps each side
Sit-ups (see page 61)	2 x 10 reps	2 x 15 reps
Back Extensions (no arms – see page 65)	2 x 10 reps	2 x 15 reps
The Plank	1 x 10 breaths	2 x 10 breaths
Sit-up and Twist (feet off floor)	1 x 20 reps each side	2 x 20 reps each side
Reverse Curls (see page 74)	1 x 20 reps	2 x 20 reps
Superman 2 (see page 69)	2 x 10 reps	2 x 16 reps
Twisting Abs (see page 75)	1 x 20 reps	2 x 20 reps

DON'T FORGET   To warm up (see pages 38–39)

SHADOW BOXING

This is an imaginary fight between you and an invisible opponent. The idea is to put together a series of punches to out-manoeuvre your imaginary sparring partner. You will probably feel silly at first dancing around the room chasing an invisible enemy but it won't be long until all is forgotten in a hail of jabs, hooks and crosses. Shadow boxing is very easy to pick up and you may be surprised how therapeutic and effective an exercise it is.

How to Make a Fist

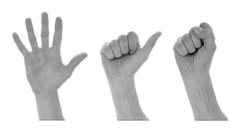

- Hold your hand out with the palm flat.
- Begin folding in from the tops of the fingers leaving out the thumb. Fold fingers over and clench them to the palm.
- Place the thumb firmly on the four folded fingers.
- Don't grip too hard.
- Avoid having long fingernails (they'll dig into your palms) and wearing rings or bracelets.

Fighting Stance

Stand sideways with your feet shoulder-width apart. Your front foot faces forward and your rear foot slightly outwards. Keep the weight distributed evenly on both legs. Make sure your knees are soft and your bodyweight is on the balls of your feet. With closed fists and bent elbows, keep your arms close to the body.

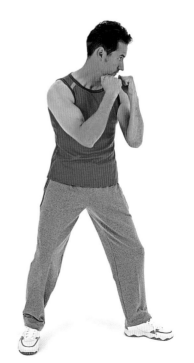

How to Punch

- Always keep your fist strong and tight but not so tense that you feel any strain in your forearm or wrist.
- Never fully extend your arm so that you are locking out any joints.
- Always give yourself a mental target when you punch.
- Remember a punch is not just thrown from the arms and shoulders; it requires the whole body mechanics behind it to be correct and to make it safe and effective.

To cool down (see pages 40–41)   To stretch (see pages 42–45)

FRONT HAND JAB ▽

The jab is a small movement. The action begins in the hips and when the punch is released the bodyweight is brought forward on to the bent front leg. Get in your fighting stance. To jab, snap the front fist out towards the target taking care not to lock out the elbow. Retract the arm quickly and return to fighting stance.

1 x 10 reps with right arm in front

1 x 10 reps with left arm in front

FRONT HOOK ▽

With the left foot leading, rotate through the ball of the left foot lifting the heel. At the same time bring the elbow of the front (left) arm in a head height 90-degree angle and drive it across the line of vision using the power from your hips. Snap back quickly to fighting stance.

1 x 10 reps with right arm in front

1 x 10 reps with left arm in front

BACK HAND CROSS ▷

Begin in fighting stance. Punch out with your back hand, pivoting on the ball of your rear foot, twisting through your waist and lifting the back heel off the floor. This is driving your bodyweight from the rear leg to the front leg. Snap the arm back to the original position.

1 x 10 reps with right arm in front

1 x 10 reps with left arm in front

DAY 18 WORKOUT

Once you have practised all three punches, start moving around in fighting stance. Try to keep light on your feet with your bodyweight forward on the ball of your foot. Do rounds of 3 minutes each throwing a combination of the above punches. Have a 1-minute break between rounds, either jogging on the spot or walking around the room. Aim to spend 20 minutes shadow boxing.

RESISTANCE WORKOUT

Today's exercises require you to lift your legs up off the floor, and hold them there during the entire move. This makes the workload for your abdominals great as it is significantly harder to control the lower body and keep it still without the lower body stability gained by having your feet on the ground. If you are in any discomfort or your legs begin to shake with the effort, drop your feet back to the floor (making sure your spine is back in a neutral position) and continue.

RAISED LEG CRUNCHES ▷

1 Lie on the floor and lift your legs up in the air. Make sure you are resting on your tailbone to protect your spine, which should be in a neutral position. Keep your knees slightly bent if you find this more comfortable, or your hamstrings (back of thighs) tight. Cup your ears with your hands.

2 Curl up from your torso bringing your head, shoulders and then shoulder blades off the floor. Rise up to an angle of about 30 degrees. Keep your chin off your chest and breathe out as you lift. Lower yourself slowly back down and repeat.

Level 1: 2 x 20 reps
Level 2: 3 x 20 reps

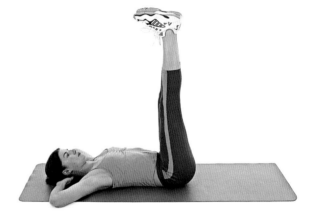

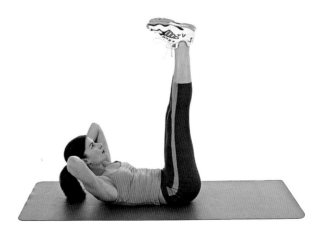

To cool down (see pages 40–41)   To stretch (see pages 42–45)

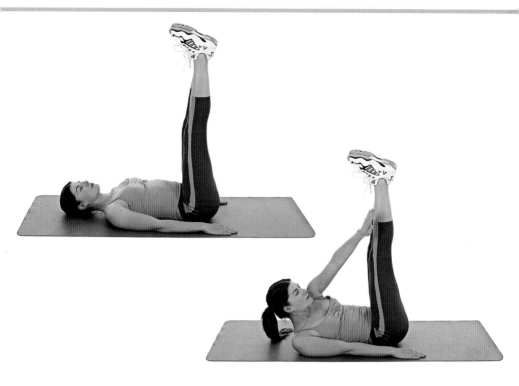

TWISTING CRUNCHES △

1 Lie down on the floor with your arms by your
sides. Lift your legs off the floor but make sure
that you are resting on your tailbone to protect your
spine, which should be in a neutral position. Keep your
knees slightly bent if you find this more comfortable.
Keep your arms flat on the floor by your sides.

2 Rise up from your torso, bringing your head,
shoulders and then shoulder blades off the floor,
twisting one arm across your body and taking it across
to the opposite knee. Breathe out as you lift up. Return
to the ground and repeat but this time taking the
other hand to the opposite knee.

Level 1: 1 x 20 reps
Level 2: 2 x 20 reps

DAY 19 WORKOUT

	Level 1	Level 2
Side Bends 2 (see page 60)	1 x 15 reps each side	2 x 15 reps each side
Raised Leg Crunches	2 x 20 reps	3 x 20 reps
Back Extensions (no arms – see page 65)	2 x 10 reps	2 x 15 reps
The Plank (see page 78)	1 x 10 breaths	2 x 10 breaths
Twisting Crunches	1 x 20 reps	2 x 20 reps
Reverse Curls (see page 74)	1 x 20 reps	2 x 20 reps
Superman 2 (see page 69)	2 x 10 reps	2 x 16 reps

RUNNING

As this is the last workout before you take a well-earned rest it is a good opportunity to make an extra effort. Instead of short bursts of running interspersed with fast walking as done on Day 9 (see pages 62–63) you will run for longer. This is not about how far you can run but how long you can keep going. The speed everyone runs at differs, and for today's exercise speed is simply not an issue.

Instead of the usual warm-up routine, an initial medium-paced walk will serve as your warm-up, while slowing down at the end will serve as a cool-down. Make sure you are wearing a watch or have a stopwatch with you.

THE WORKOUT

1 Begin by starting with a medium-paced walk, then over the first 10 minutes build up gradually to a fast-paced walk.

2 When you have completed your 10-minute walking warm-up, break into a slow jog and spend the next 10–20 minutes jogging or running at a comfortable pace.

3 Finish with a 10-minute cool-down walk. Start slowing the pace of your jogging down before you break into a very brisk walk. Over the 10-minute period gradually slow down to a medium-paced walk, letting your heart rate and breathing return to normal.

If you really enjoy running, consider taking it up more seriously. There are many clubs available for all levels from beginners upwards, and not only will they help you improve your running abilities, but they are also a great way to meet like-minded people.

You might even think about entering yourself in a local marathon – it is not as tough as it sounds. Many start at as little a distance as 5 km (3 miles) and build up from there. It is a great way to focus on improving your running.

Running at Night

• Wear reflective clothing. You need to be seen by other road users. Many trainers do have reflective strips, but it is also advisable to buy some reflective strips to wear over your exercise clothes.
• Walk or run facing oncoming traffic so you can see where you are going and be seen by oncoming cars.
• If you are running on the pavement, have some respect for your fellow pedestrians. It can be quite alarming if someone runs up behind you out of nowhere, so do let them know you are coming.
• Exercise with a friend or let someone know your running route for safety.

TECHNIQUE POINTS

• Keep your feet close to the ground.

• Land on your heels, then roll through the whole of the foot.

• Relax your shoulders and hands – don't tense them into fists.

To cool down (see pages 40–41)   To stretch (see pages 42–45)

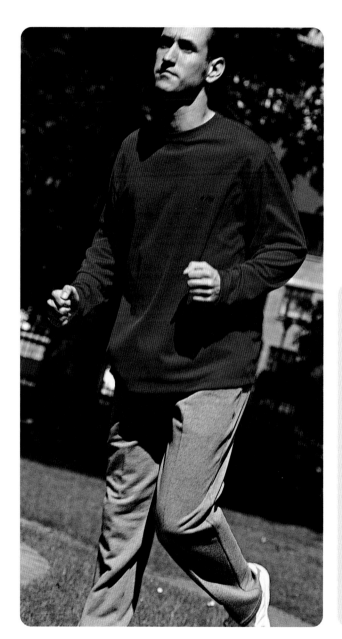

TIPS

- If you feel out of breath during your jog or run, either slow down the pace or break into a fast walk until you have recovered.
- Don't be put off by other joggers running past you. You are not competing in a race.
- Don't try too hard. It is tempting to charge off at too fast a pace. This will only make you out of breath much more quickly.
- Don't daydream – keep an eye on where you are running. Look out for broken paving stones, kerbs or uneven terrain.

REST DAY

This is your last rest day of the 30-day programme. As you have done on other rest days, spend some time revisiting your original goals and, if you feel that you have drifted away from any of the plan, use them to help you get back on track. The days ahead are going to be tough, but having made it this far you are more than capable of doing what is required.

Make sure you make use of visualization techniques and positive reinforcement. Imagine yourself feeling happy with your new improved body, which is now so strong and supple. Tear out a few pictures from magazines of how you would like to look and stick them up in obvious places, such as on the fridge door or food cupboards as a source of constant motivation. Finally, stand naked in front of the mirror and admire the difference you have made already to your body – just nine more days left!

Some form of pampering is entirely appropriate on your rest day. Self-massage has been around in eastern traditions for centuries, and with good reason. Why not focus on an extremely hard-working but often overlooked part of the body: the feet? A relaxing foot massage will be particularly welcome after yesterday's running. If you have never done one before, simply wash your feet, then follow the directions given below. Or, for a real treat, book a session with a professional practitioner.

JAPANESE SHIATSU TREATMENT FOR FEET

1 Press each toe hard 3 times with your thumb, working down from the tips of the toes to the foot itself.

2 Now press between the tendons on the top of the foot, grasping the foot in your hand and working up between each tendon towards the ankle.

3 Move to the sole of the foot (the plantar arch), pressing hard with your thumb on the bottom of the foot, moving up towards the centre.

4 Finally, apply firm pressure around the sides of the ankles and the Achilles tendon.

5 Repeat on the other foot, then put your feet up on a cushion so your legs and feet are above the level of your head and body, and relax with your eyes closed for at least 5 minutes.

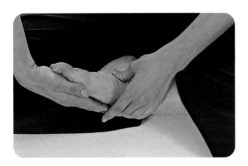

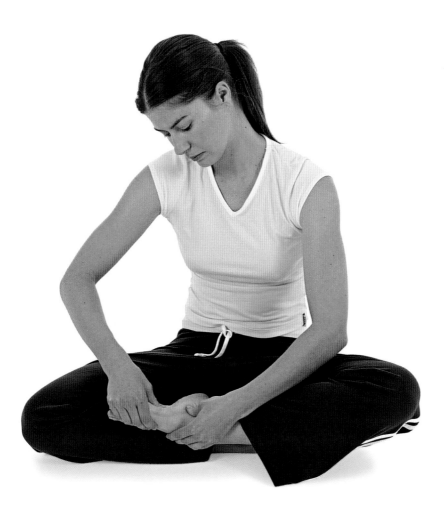

RESISTANCE WORKOUT

You will be using a stability (Swiss) ball today to help target your core stability muscles (see page 14). The ball makes you work much harder as the rest of your body has to work hard at keeping the ball in place while you carry out the exercise.

Ball work can also improve posture. Anyone sitting at a desk who is prone to lower-back pain due to poor posture could substitute a ball for the chair. As the ball doesn't have a supporting back, you have to work harder at keeping your body upright, rather than slumping into the back of a chair. Note, however, that this whole body adjustment will take some time, so alternate between the ball and the chair to begin with.

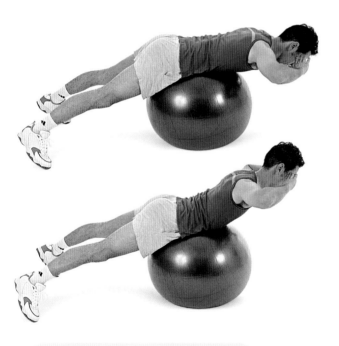

BACK EXTENSIONS (OFF BALL) ◁

1 Kneel down facing the ball and push yourself up on top so the ball is underneath the abdominals. Plant your feet shoulder-width apart resting on your toes with a slight bend in the knee. Place your fingertips next to your temples and roll your chest over the front of the ball.

2 Lift your chest so that your back is straight, but not arched. Keep your head neutral (neither dropping your chin forward nor raising it up) and look at the floor throughout the exercise.

Level 1: 2 x 20 reps
Level 2: 3 x 20 reps

TECHNIQUE POINT
• If you find it difficult to balance, keep your knees on the floor. This may limit your range of movement.

To cool down (see pages 40–41)   To stretch (see pages 42–45)

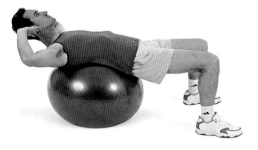

AB CURLS (OFF BALL) ◁

1 Sit on the ball and walk yourself forward so that the ball sits in the curve of your lower back. Keep your feet flat on the floor and your knees bent at 90 degrees. Cup your ears with your hands, letting your elbows fall naturally out.

2 Now slowly roll your shoulders forwards and push your bottom into the ball. Lower yourself back down so your back is straight.

Level 1: 2 x 20 reps
Level 2: 3 x 20 reps

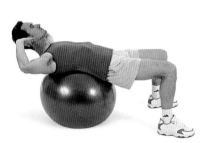

DAY 22 WORKOUT

	Level 1	Level 2
Side Bends 2 (see page 60)	1 x 15 reps each side	2 x 15 reps each side
Raised Leg Crunches (see page 82)	2 x 20 reps	3 x 20 reps
Back Extensions (off ball)	2 x 20 reps	3 x 20 reps
Ab Curls (off ball)	2 x 20 reps	3 x 20 reps
The Plank (see page 78)	1 x 10 breaths	2 x 10 breaths
Twisting Crunches (see page 83)	1 x 20 reps	2 x 20 reps
Superman 2 (see page 69)	2 x 10 reps	2 x 16 reps
Reverse Curls (see page 74)	1 x 20 reps	2 x 20 reps

TECHNIQUE POINTS

• Remember to breathe out as you lift up.

• Keep a gap between your chin and your chest. Imagine you are holding an orange or tennis ball in place.

PLYOMETRIC WORKOUT 1

Today's workout includes some old-fashioned playground favourites such as hopping, skipping and jumping. Known as plyometrics, this is a great way to improve the power and efficiency of all muscle groups and to work on your cardiovascular fitness. A slightly soft surface, such as grass or a sprung floor, is preferable to help minimize the impact on your joints, but you can do it at home – indoors or outdoors.

Begin as always with your warm-up and then add on another 5 minutes of gentle jogging. In between each of the following moves spend 2 minutes jogging or walking around to help you recover from the workout. Explosive movements are the key to optimum results and do make sure you keep your technique as perfect as possible. Use only your bodyweight and aim to stay on the ball of your foot whenever possible.

BOUNDS ▷

1 This move involves the same movement as your natural running action, but in an exaggerated form. Push off from your right leg and drive your left knee forwards and upwards as if kicking a football.

2 Land on your left foot and push off, this time driving your right knee forwards and upwards. Use your arms to help maintain balance and power.

Level 1: 1 x 10 reps
Level 2: 2 x 10 reps

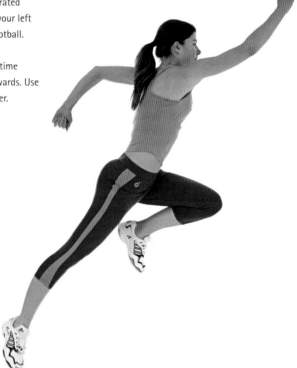

To cool down (see pages 40–41)   To stretch (see pages 42–45)

HOPS ▷

Start this exercise using your stronger leg. Bend it slightly and push off forcefully to spring forward. Try to keep the upper body straight and try not to twist through the waist. Keep the opposite knee as high as you can, and use your arms to propel yourself forwards. Land flat-footed with the knee slightly bent, repeat, then do the same with the other leg.

Level 1: 1 x 10 reps each leg
Level 2: 2 x 10 reps each leg

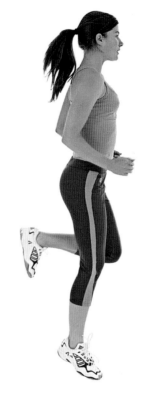

SQUAT THRUSTS ▽

1 Place your hands on the floor, shoulder-width apart, with your fingers pointing forwards. Take your legs back until your body is almost in a straight line.

2 Now, jump forwards with both feet, bringing your knees in towards your chest. As soon as you land, jump back to the starting position and repeat. Remember to keep your abdominal muscles tight throughout the move and your buttocks low – don't stick them up in the air!

Level 1: 1 x 10 reps
Level 2: 2 x 10 reps

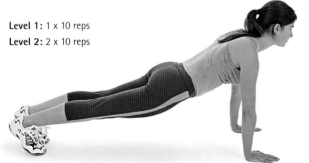
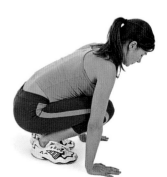

DON'T FORGET   To warm up (see pages 38–39)

RESISTANCE WORKOUT

You are back on the stability ball for today's workout. Remember that it is important to make sure the ball retains its original firmness by using the pump provided when necessary.

You can use your ball during non-exercise times, too. Try reading or watching television while sitting on it – it is a great way to help improve your posture without really trying.

OBLIQUE CURLS ▷

1 Sit on the ball and walk yourself forwards so the ball sits in the curve of your lower back. Keep your knees bent at a 90-degree angle with your feet flat on the floor. Cup your ears with your hands letting your elbows fall naturally out.

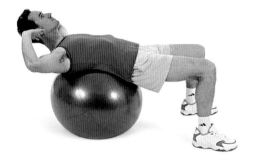

2 Slowly roll your shoulders forwards and take one shoulder towards the opposite knee. Lower yourself back down so your back is straight. Perform the required number of repetitions and then change sides.

Level 1: 1 x 20 reps
Level 2: 2 x 20 reps

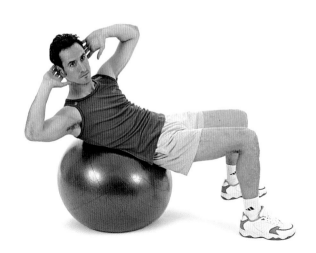

To cool down (see pages 40–41)   To stretch (see pages 42–45)

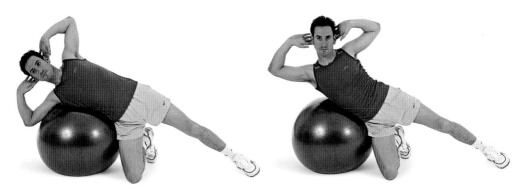

LATERAL CRUNCHES △

1 Kneel by the side of the ball with your hip resting against it. Roll yourself on to the ball so that your hip now rests on it and you can lie over the ball on your side. Keep the lower knee on the floor and extend the top knee so it is almost straight. Place your fingertips at your temples and keep a gap between your chin and your chest.

2 Keeping the body straight, lift yourself up so that your uppermost elbow moves towards the hip of the outstretched leg. Allow your body to lower back over the ball and repeat.

Level 1: 1 x 20 reps each side
Level 2: 2 x 20 reps each side

TECHNIQUE POINT
• This exercise requires a lot of balance. It can be made easier by bracing your feet against a wall. Keep your body in a straight line from head to toe. When lifting, don't let your back rotate.

DAY 24 WORKOUT

	Level 1	Level 2
Raised Leg Crunches (see page 82)	2 x 20 reps	3 x 20 reps
Ab Curls (off ball – see page 89)	2 x 20 reps	3 x 20 reps
Back Extensions (off ball – see page 88)	2 x 20 reps	3 x 20 reps
Oblique Curls	1 x 20 reps	2 x 20 reps
Lateral Crunches	1 x 20 reps each side	2 x 20 reps each side
Superman 2 (see page 69)	2 x 10 reps	2 x 16 reps
Reverse Curls (see page 74)	1 x 20 reps	2 x 20 reps

FARTLEK WORKOUT

Fartlek is a Swedish word that is roughly translated as 'speed-play'. This form of training involves practising a combination of varied pace running – for example, interrupting a steady jog to break into a short fast sprint. It is an extremely effective way of helping to improve anyone's cardiovascular abilities and it will also burn off a significant number of calories. It is best to do this workout on grass if possible.

You do not need to follow the original warm-up routine in this instance. Instead, spend the first 5 minutes building up from a medium pace to a brisk walk, and then continue with the exercises shown below.

JOGGING (5 MINUTES)

Begin the workout with an even-paced 5-minute jog. Use this as an extension to your warm-up walk to prepare the body for the harder work to come.

MEDIUM-PACED RUN (3 MINUTES)

After your initial 5-minute jog, move up a gear to a medium-paced run. You should still be able to breathe relatively easily at the beginning of the 3 minutes but should be finding it progressively more difficult towards the end. If, however, you find yourself getting out of breath too quickly, slow the pace down a notch.

BRISK WALK (2 MINUTES)

You should be breathing heavily at the end of the medium-paced run so use this brisk walk as a recovery phase. Make sure you do walk briskly for the entire 2 minutes. Stride out and use your arms to propel yourself forwards.

MEDIUM-PACED RUN WITH SPRINTS (5 MINUTES)

Take yourself back up into a medium-paced run. Every 200 m (220 yards), sprint for 50–60 m (55–65 yards). Use natural landmarks such as benches or trees to mark your short sprints.

JOGGING (2 MINUTES)

The medium-paced run with sprints should leave you breathing heavily or even out of breath. The 2-minute jogging phase is intended to help you recover your breath in readiness for the final hard section to come.

JOGGING WITH FAST RUNS (4 MINUTES)

Continue jogging, then speed up to a fast run for 20–30 m (22–33 yards) after 2 minutes. Return to a jog, then repeat after the next 2 minutes. This is the last (and one of the hardest) sections of your workout so do give it your all. You should be feeling tired so now is the time to pull out all the stops for your last fast runs. It will all be worth it!

JOGGING (2 MINUTES)

Take the pace down now towards your final cool-down section. Allow your breathing to slow down for you to recover but keep the jog at an even pace.

BRISK WALK (5 MINUTES)

Use the last 5 minutes' brisk walk to cool down and allow your breathing and heart rate to return to normal. Do not be tempted to suddenly stop. This is an important stage as you must allow your body to return slowly and safely to its pre-exercise state.

To cool down (see pages 40–41)   To stretch (see pages 42–45)

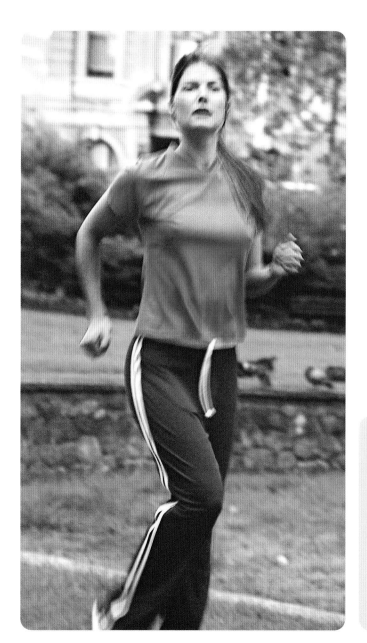

TIP
• Make sure you finish this workout with a good all-over stretch, concentrating especially on your calves, hamstrings, hip flexors and front of thighs.

RESISTANCE WORKOUT

Today's session contains one of the most difficult exercises for the abdominal muscles, The Oblique Bridge. Hard as it is, the results are certainly worth it – you can achieve a very sculpted and lean-looking waistline in double-quick time. Make sure, with both of the new exercises today, you use focus and control – you are an experienced exerciser now but even the best can make mistakes, allowing concentration to slip from time to time.

THE OBLIQUE BRIDGE ▷

1 Lie on your side and position your elbow directly under your shoulder as support.

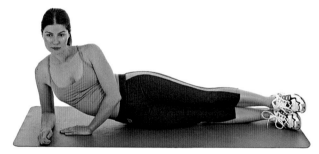

2 Place one foot on top of the other, then raise yourself up, keeping a straight line from your head to your toes. Hold this position by tightening your obliques (the muscles at the side of your stomach that run from your ribcage to your hips). Hold for the requisite breaths and then lower yourself slowly down. Do not hold your breath at any point. Repeat on the other side.

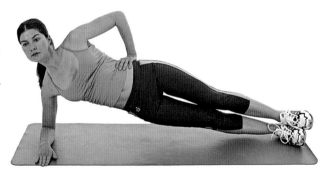

Level 1: 1 x 5 breaths each side
Level 2: 2 x 5 breaths each side

To cool down (see pages 40–41)   To stretch (see pages 42–45)

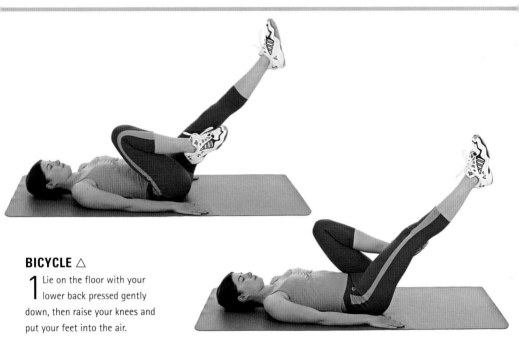

BICYCLE △

1 Lie on the floor with your lower back pressed gently down, then raise your knees and put your feet into the air.

2 Rotate your legs as though you were cycling, pressing through a softly flexed foot. Make sure that you do not twist or raise your back and keep your abdominals tight at all times.

Level 1: 1 x 20 reps
Level 2: 2 x 20 reps

DAY 26 WORKOUT

	Level 1	Level 2
Raised Leg Crunches (see page 82)	2 x 20 reps	3 x 20 reps
The Oblique Bridge	1 x 5 breaths each side	2 x 5 breaths each side
Bicycle	1 x 20 reps	2 x 20 reps
Back Extensions (off ball – see page 88)	2 x 20 reps	3 x 20 reps
Ab Curls (off ball – see page 89)	2 x 20 reps	3 x 20 reps
Superman 2 (see page 69)	2 x 10 reps	2 x 16 reps
The Plank (see page 78)	1 x 10 breaths	2 x 10 breaths

TECHNIQUE POINT

• Start with your feet directly above the line of your hips. To make this harder drop the line of the legs towards the floor keeping your back firmly on the ground at all times.

PLYOMETRIC WORKOUT 2

Today you are revisiting a plyometric workout similar to the one first featured on Day 23 (see pages 90–91). Remember to use your normal warm-up and then add on 5 minutes of gentle jogging to make sure your body is thoroughly warmed up. In between each of the following moves do 2 minutes of walking or jogging around to help you recover.

BUNNY HOPS ▷

Stand with your feet shoulder-width apart. Bend your knees slightly and then spring forwards and upwards as far and as high as you can, bringing your knees in towards your chest. Try to keep your back straight – don't bend forwards – and swing your arms upwards as you jump. Keep your abdominal muscles tight. Land flat-footed on both feet, bending the knees on landing to help cushion the impact. From this semi-squat position, spring up again and repeat the movement for the required repetitions.

Level 1: 1 x 10 hops
Level 2: 2 x 10 hops

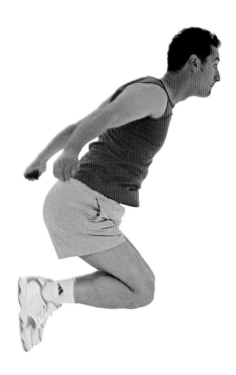

TECHNIQUE POINT
• The aim is to keep going and not stop between bunny hops, so maintain the momentum.

To cool down (see pages 40–41)   To stretch (see pages 42–45)

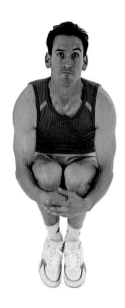

TUCK JUMPS ◁

Start with your feet hip-width apart, abdominals tight and your back straight. Jump up high while trying to tuck both knees into your chest. Land as softly as possible, sinking into the knees and ankles. Jump straight back up.

Level 1: 1 x 5 jumps
Level 2: 1 x 10 jumps

ASTRIDE JUMPS ▷

These are similar to the bunny hops, but this time you are going from side to side. Start by marking out on the ground a 20–30 cm (8–12 in) space that you are going to jump over (you can increase this as you improve). Begin on one side with your feet hip-width apart and your knees slightly bent. Spring sideways over your marker landing flat-footed and bending at the knees to help soften the impact. Spring immediately back over.

Level 1: 1 x 10 jumps
Level 2: 2 x 10 jumps

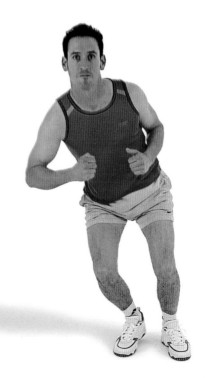

RESISTANCE WORKOUT

Boxing and martial arts are the inspiration for today's two new exercises. By incorporating a Front Hook punch from Day 18 (see page 81) into a sit-up you are working not only your abdominals but also your waist. The Twister requires the use of your now much-improved abdominal muscles to hold you firmly in place while your waist does the work.

SIT-UP AND HOOK ▷

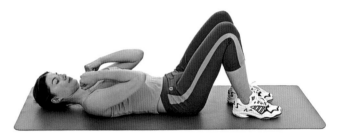

1 Lie on your back with your knees bent and your feet flat on the floor. Gently press your lower back into a neutral spine position. Making soft fists, bend your elbows bringing the arms up towards your chest. Lift through the head and shoulders then the shoulder blades, squeezing through the abdominals, while coming up as high as feels comfortable.

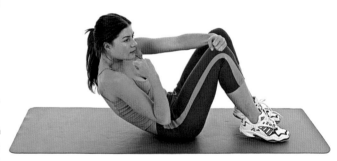

2 As you reach the top of the movement throw a right hook, immediately followed by a left one. Keep the pace slow to medium, breathing out as you punch. Return to the ground and repeat, this time throwing a left hook first, followed by a right, and so on.

Level 1: 1 x 20 reps
Level 2: 2 x 20 reps

TECHNIQUE POINT

• Make sure the work comes from the waist, while the pelvis remains steadfastly on the floor.

To cool down (see pages 40–41)   To stretch (see pages 42–45)

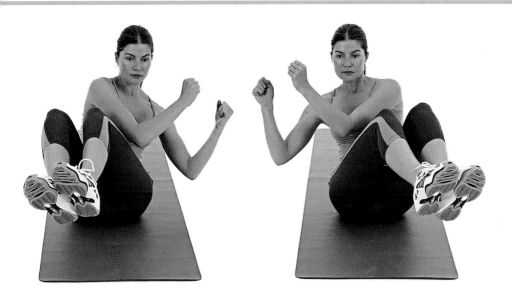

THE TWISTER △

1 Sit with your knees bent and back straight. Now, lifting your knees directly off the ground and keeping your knees slightly bent, find the balance point on your lower sacrum (the bottom section of vertebrae in your back).

2 Keeping the abdominal muscles tight, begin to twist from side to side. Concentrate on working through the waist and on keeping your balance. Breathe out as you twist.

Level 1: 2 x 10 twists
Level 2: 2 x 20 twists

DAY 28 WORKOUT

	Level 1	Level 2
Raised Leg Crunches (see page 82)	2 x 20 reps	3 x 20 reps
The Oblique Bridge (see page 96)	1 x 5 breaths each side	2 x 5 breaths each side
Back Extensions (off ball – see page 88)	2 x 20 reps	3 x 20 reps
Sit-up and Hook	1 x 20 reps	2 x 20 reps
Superman 2 (see page 69)	2 x 10 reps	2 x 16 reps
The Twister	2 x 10 twists	2 x 20 twists
The Plank (see page 78)	1 x 10 breaths	2 x 10 breaths
Reverse Curls (see page 74)	1 x 20 reps	2 x 20 reps

DON'T FORGET To warm up (see pages 38–39)

AEROBIC CIRCUIT

By now you should be feeling – and looking – fantastic. As this is your penultimate day of the 30-day programme, you may feel that there is nothing else you can do to make a difference in the last couple of days, but rest assured that every little thing will make a difference. So keep concentrating and try to keep your enthusiasm high. Really enjoy today's aerobic component; remember how hard you have worked to reached this level of fitness.

Spend 2 minutes completing each of these 'aerobic stations', with no rest between. Try to do 4 circuits, so that you complete each station 4 times. If you feel yourself getting out of breath, walk or jog through it until you have recovered sufficiently to continue with the next station.

STEP ▷

Step up and down on the step 10 times leading with your left leg, followed by 10 with the right leg. Keep repeating this pattern for the whole 2 minutes. Make sure you put your whole foot on the step and stand up straight. Keep your abdominals tight. Punch your arms out in front, but take care not to lock out the elbows. Repeat for 2 minutes.

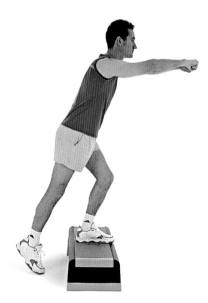

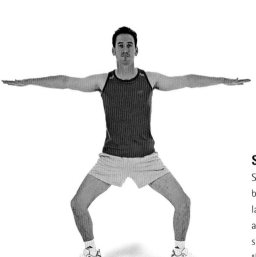

STAR JUMPS ◁

Start with your feet hip-width apart and your arms by your sides. Slightly bend the knees and jump out, landing with your feet one-and-a-half times hip-width apart. Make sure you land with slightly bent knees, sinking into the move to absorb the excess impact. At the same time lift your arms out to the side moving up to above your head. Immediately jump back to the start position and repeat for 2 minutes.

To cool down (see pages 40–41)   To stretch (see pages 42–45)

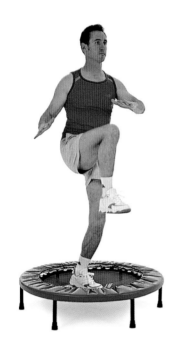

KNEE LIFTS ◁

Standing on the rebounder, bring the opposite hand to the opposite knee so you are doing knee lifts. Keep your back straight and your abdominals tight. Keep the supporting knee slightly bent at all times. Continue for 2 minutes.

SKIPPING

Stand upright and keep your abdominal muscles tight. Hold the rope with your hands out to the side and your elbows in. Push off with the balls of your feet to jump. Don't jump too high and keep your knees slightly bent. Keep going for 2 minutes.

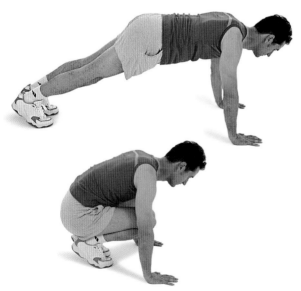

SQUAT THRUSTS ◁

Place your hands on the floor, shoulder-width apart with your fingers pointing forwards. Take your legs back until your body is almost in a straight line. Now, jump forwards with both feet, bringing your knees in towards your chest. As soon as you land, jump straight back to the starting position and repeat for 2 minutes.

ALTERNATIVE WORKOUT

Do a 45-minute walk or run at 80 per cent MHR (see page 35).

Day 30

GRAND FINALE

You have come a long way since Day 1! You have adopted some admirable new habits in the form of daily exercise and healthy eating, and consequently lost inches and now have a flatter tummy. Keep up the good work by following the maintenance advice that follows in the next chapter (see pages 106–115).

But first, make yourself proud today by finishing your 30-day programme with an extra-special workout. It incorporates both boxing and abdominal toning, giving you a cardiovascular resistance programme that should leave you glowing not just with the effort of hard work but also with pride.

DAY 30 WORKOUT

		Level 1	Level 2
	Ab Curls (off ball) (see page 89)	2 x 20 reps	3 x 20 reps
	Shadow Boxing (see pages 80–81)	3 minutes	3 minutes
	Oblique Curls (see page 92)	2 x 20 reps	3 x 20 reps
	Shadow Boxing (see pages 80–81)	3 minutes	3 minutes

To cool down (see pages 40–41)   To stretch (see pages 42–45)

		Level 1	Level 2
Back Extensions (off ball) (see page 88)		2 x 20 reps	3 x 20 reps
Shadow Boxing (see pages 80–81)		3 minutes	3 minutes
Lateral Crunches (see page 93)		1 x 20 reps each side	2 x 20 reps each side
The Plank (see page 78)		2 x 10 breaths	3 x 10 breaths
Superman 2 (see page 69)		1 x 20 reps	2 x 20 reps
Sit-up and Hook (see page 100)		1 x 20 reps	2 x 20 reps
Reverse Curls (see page 74)		1 x 20 reps	2 x 20 reps

Keeping Your New Body Shape

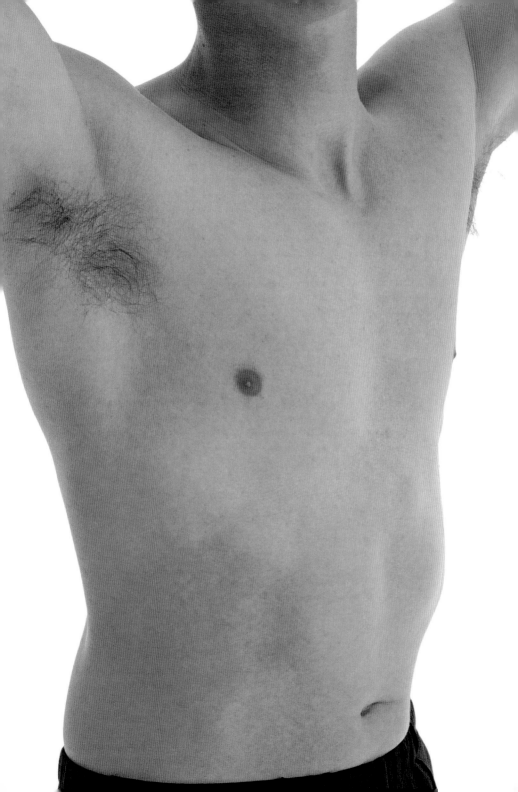

Body Maintenance

Congratulations on completing the 30-day programme! Now is the time to fill in the final column of your Body Measurements Chart (see page 21) and to savour your success. As you will be aware, it is the result of two things: eating more healthily and a regime of daily exercise.

Maintaining your new body shape will depend on keeping up these admirable new habits and this chapter aims to help you achieve that. It contains tips on continuing to eat well as well as some ideas for fitness programmes to follow in the future.

LONG-TERM HEALTHY EATING

If your initial aim over the last 30 days was not only to tone your tummy but to lose excess weight, then you should have been cutting your food intake by 400–500 calories a day to aid fat loss. It is the consumption of fewer daily calories combined with increased levels of exercise that has helped you reach your goal.

But what happens from here? This depends on whether you have reached your initial weight-loss goal. If you have, then you can begin to relax your diet and exercise programme to a degree. However, if you have a few excess pounds to go, then it is advisable to carry on cutting out those extra calories for a little while longer.

Maintaining your weight loss and new-found figure should be a more relaxed affair, though this doesn't mean that you can slip back into old bad habits. Try to eat as healthily as possible in general but allow yourself an occasional treat. One method that works for many people is to allow yourself one day a week when you eat pretty much what you feel like (within reason!) and do not feel guilty about it. You may prefer a couple of treats a week slotted in at random. Find a method of treating yourself without going overboard – and then stick to it. Finally, follow the Golden Rules (see opposite) to help you maintain your new shape.

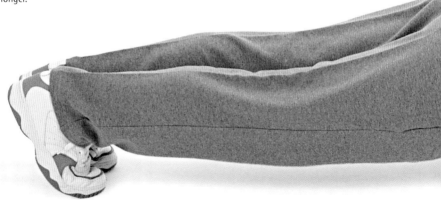

GOLDEN RULES OF HEALTHY EATING

1 Eat breakfast every day and continue to have three meals a day with small healthy snacks in between. Remember that eating little and often will boost your metabolism, keep you fuelled and therefore less tempted to eat unhealthy foods.

2 Don't let old bad habits return when you are doing your food shopping. Plan the weekly menu in advance and shop accordingly. Resist the temptation to restock the cupboards with junk food and snacks.

3 Be careful not to become too complacent over time. If you find that you have slipped back into bad habits, make a conscious effort to improve your diet – it may help you to write another food diary (see page 29). If necessary, do the 30-day programme over again.

4 Remember that there is still plenty of scope to enjoy cooking and eating healthily. Food is supposed to be fun!

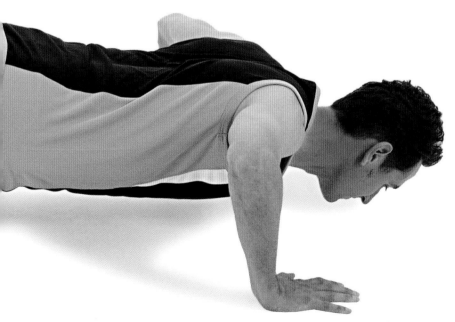

Maintenance Exercises

You have worked very hard over the last 30 days and now it is time for you to begin maintaining your new-found fitness. As with your daily diet there are a few rules you need to follow in order to stop you slipping back into those pre-exercise days. Rest assured that maintenance exercise won't be as intensive as the last 30 days, but it will be as effective.

DAILY EXERCISE

Try to do some form of aerobic exercise at least once a day. It doesn't need to be formal exercise but do look at your lifestyle and find ways to increase activity within it. Spending as little as 15 minutes daily working your cardiovascular system will make a huge long-term difference not just to your weight stability but to your health in general. Here are some ideas for leading a more active lifestyle:
• Take the stairs instead of a lift or escalator.
• Don't use the car for short journeys – always walk.
• Involve your family in healthy activities – bike riding, swimming and walking are excellent ways for all to get fit and share some quality family time.
• Find hobbies that keep you fit – try skating or dancing or take up a sport.

In addition to increased daily activity try to do some organized exercise 3 times a week for a minimum of 30 minutes. Cardiovascular work will help burn calories and maintain a healthy heart and lungs (aim to get sweaty and out of breath). General muscle toning will stop you looking flabby and keep that tummy in check. Ideally, as in the 30-day programme, aim to do a combination of both.

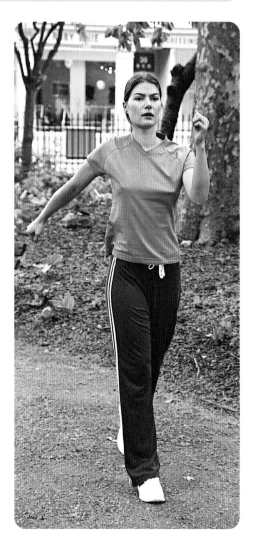

CROSS TRAINING

A valuable tip for maintaining long-term health and fitness is to keep motivated by trying new forms of exercise. The body can become complacent when doing the same routine week in and week out. This is called 'plateau-ing', and can be diagnosed when however hard you work you do not get the same results. Cross training – varying your routine over time – is the key to ongoing success. Try some of the following forms of exercise.

Running

Running is a great way to keep fit and meet like-minded people. Did your taste of some of the many different forms over the last 30 days spark your interest? Try cross-country running or join one of the many running clubs catering to people of all levels. Why not sign up for one of the many mini-marathons open to non-professionals world-wide?

Swimming

Even if you are not a strong swimmer do consider this as an option for part of your on-going cross-training programme. Swimming is a fantastic all-over body workout, which is relatively cheap and convenient for most people.

Cycling

As with running this is a sport that not only keeps you fit but can also be done alone or in the company of others. Look out for local clubs in your nearest cycle shop or the telephone directory. If you are one of the many people who have bikes rusting away somewhere, it is well worth spending some money getting your bike thoroughly overhauled by a professional.

Weight Training

Not just for the muscle-bound, weight training – properly used – can keep you firm and toned for life and help keep that excess fat from building up again. Combine it with a simple aerobic programme and you are on to a winner.

Exercise to Music Classes

These classes come in many guises these days, giving you many interesting options. Most local health clubs and leisure centres offer choices from simple aerobics, through step aerobics to body toning classes. Try as many differing styles as possible to find out which suits you best.

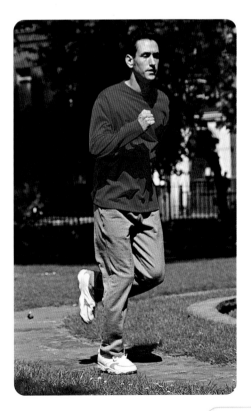

Weekly Exercise Plan

To keep up your exercising in the long term, you should choose at least three out of the following six workouts to fit into your week. Aim to exercise for 30 minutes, and don't forget to warm up (see pages 38-39), cool down (see pages 40-41) and stretch (see pages 42-45) properly. You should avoid doing the more strenuous workouts (1-4) on consecutive days, but you can do any of the exercises in workout 6 (see page 115) at any point during the week.

WORKOUT 1
Abdominal Routine

	Level 1	Level 2
Warm-up (see pages 38-39)		
Sit-ups (see page 61)	2 x 20 reps	3 x 20 reps
Superman 2 (see page 69)	2 x 20 reps	3 x 20 reps
Sit-up and Twist (feet off floor – see page 79)	2 x 20 reps	3 x 20 reps
The Plank (see page 78)	2 x 10 breaths	3 x 10 breaths
Back Extensions (no arms – see page 65)	2 x 20 reps	3 x 20 reps
Stretches (see page 42-45)		

You could also choose any of the other resistance routines from the 30-day programme (see the odd days: Day 1, Day 3, etc.) and do five of these in addition to warm-up and cool-down exercises.

WORKOUT 2

This is an all-over body workout to do at the gym. It is very important to make sure you are shown how to use all gym equipment by a trained professional. Ask for advice in setting specific weights, sets and repetitions.

1 Start with a 20-minute aerobic workout, which can consist of brisk walking, running, cycling or rowing.

2 Follow with a resistance workout on the weight machines:
Leg Press: Leg Extensions and Leg Curls.
Bench Press: Lateral Pulldowns.
Shoulder Press: Basic Sit-ups and Back Extensions.
End with an **all-over body stretch** (see pages 42-45).

WORKOUT 3

This routine can be done at home. Some of the exercises use hand weights weighing about 2 kg (4 lb). Squats work the front of your thighs and your buttocks; the Tricep Dips work your chest, backs of arms and the front of your shoulders; the One-arm Rows work your back and your biceps and the Lateral Raises work your shoulders.

SQUATS ▽

1 Stand with your feet one-and-half times hip-width apart, feet facing forwards or pointing slightly outwards.

2 Squat down by flexing the knees and hips making sure your back stays straight throughout. Keep your head facing forwards and the abdominals tight. Squat to a position where your thighs are roughly parallel to the ground – don't go lower than this. Straighten up back to the start position, making sure you do not lock out your knee joints at the top of the move. Repeat immediately.

Level 1: 2 x 15 reps
Level 2: 2 x 20 reps

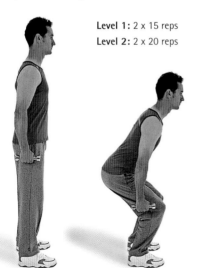

TRICEP DIPS ▽

1 Sit on the edge of a stable chair and place your hands on the chair at either side of your upper thighs, fingers pointing forwards. Your legs are at right angles and hip-width apart. Keeping your legs in the same position shuffle off the chair taking your bodyweight on to your arms. At this point your arms should be straight but not locked out.

2 Flex at the elbows and lower your buttocks towards the floor. Keep your back close to the chair and your abdominal muscles tight. Don't flex the elbows to more than 90 degrees. Straighten up to the start position again taking care not to lock out your elbows. Repeat immediately.

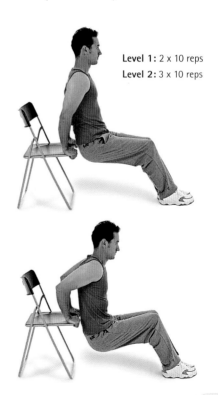

Level 1: 2 x 10 reps
Level 2: 3 x 10 reps

ONE-ARM ROWS ▷

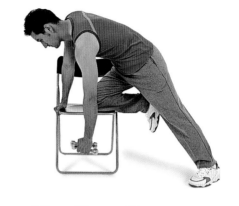

1 Use a stable chair or bench. Place your right hand and knee on the chair. The left foot on the floor forms the third point of a triangular stable base. This leg should be slightly bent and comfortable. Keep your back straight and look forward and down. Extend your left arm and grasp hold of both of your hand weights in your left hand.

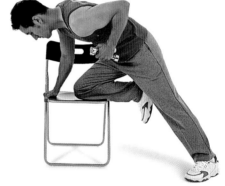

2 Keeping your left wrist straight and leading with your elbow, draw the hand weights up to your armpit keeping your arm close to your body. Straighten your arm slowly back to the start position taking care not to lock out your elbow. Repeat.

Level 1: 2 x 10 reps
Level 2: 3 x 10 reps

LATERAL RAISES ▽

1 Stand with your feet one-and-a-half times hip-width apart, buttocks tucked under and your knees slightly bent. Hold your hand weights by your sides with your palms facing in. Bend the arms slightly and keep the wrists straight.

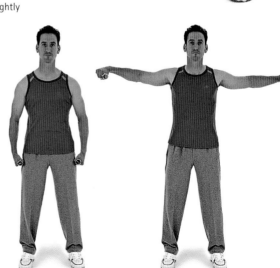

2 Raise the weights out to the side leading the movement with your knuckles while keeping a slight bend in your elbows. Take your arms up to shoulder height and then lower back slowly under control. Repeat.

Level 1: 2 x 10 reps
Level 2: 3 x 10 reps

ALL-OVER BODY STRETCH

See pages 42–45.

WORKOUT 4

Choose any of the aerobic workouts from the 30-day programme (see the even-numbered days: Day 2, Day 4, etc.) and do the whole thing.

WORKOUT 5

This workout is a weekend winner. Any of the following activities are perfect for doing over the weekend. Get family or friends to join in to make it even more fun.

• 30-minute swimming session.
• 30–60-minute brisk cross-country walk.
• 30–60-minute cycle ride.
• Exercise to music class.
• Aerobic video.
• 30 minutes' dancing.
• 30 minutes' ice-skating, roller-blading or horse-riding.
• 30 minutes' playing football or rounders with friends or family.

WORKOUT 6 ▷

Fit these activities into your daily routine whenever you can:

• Walk to or from work.
• Cycle to work or the shops.
• Only take the stairs all day.
• Do 10 minutes on the rebounder.
• Take the dog and/or children for a fast walk.
• Spend 5–10 minutes walking or jogging up and down stairs.
• Take a 10-minute jog around the block.
• Do 10 minutes' skipping with a skipping rope.

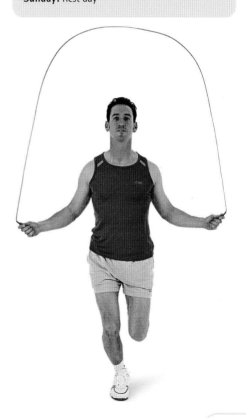

SAMPLE WEEKLY WORKOUT

It is a good idea to plan your week in advance so that you are less likely to miss a day's exercise. A well-structured weekly workout would be something like this:

Monday: Rest day
Tuesday: Workout 2 (all-over body workout)
Wednesday: Rest day
Thursday: Workout 1 (abdominal routine)
Friday: Workout 6 (in-between workout)
Saturday: Workout 5 (weekend winner)
Sunday: Rest day

Pre- and Post-Natal Exercises

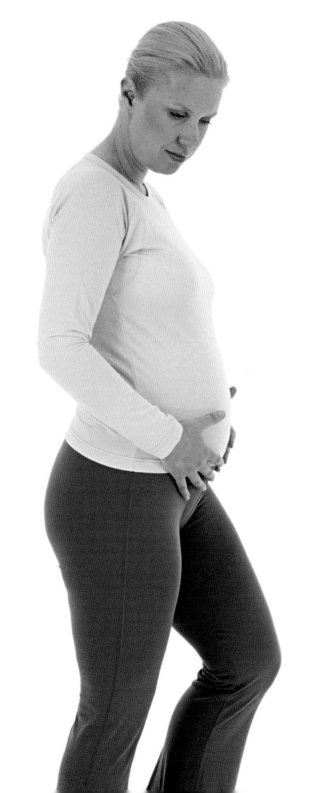

Exercising During Pregnancy

Being pregnant itself is a daily workout and, as the months progress, even the simplest tasks can become strenuous. Of course, this isn't everybody's experience; a lucky few manage to sail through the whole nine months feeling on top of the world. There are ways, however, that you can tip the balance in your favour and consistent exercise is one of them.

Research has shown that exercise during pregnancy can make the mother feel more comfortable, shorten labour and reduce the need for obstetric interventions. According to one study, regular exercise appears to improve not only physical fitness but also all-round feelings of positive body image – quite an important issue for many pregnant women.

A CHANGE IN EMPHASIS

Understandably, exercising during pregnancy is different to working out normally. The whole emphasis should change from improving your fitness levels to maintaining them. This is not the time to lose weight or begin a vigorous exercise routine. Now is the time to keep up your fitness levels and help improve specifically important areas, such as your pelvic floor muscles, which can become severely weakened during pregnancy and labour.

There are various factors to be taken into consideration. If you had a sedentary lifestyle before you were pregnant, it is vital that you review any

possible exercise plan with your healthcare provider before you begin. Nonetheless, if you aren't in any of the high-risk categories (see below), you can pursue an exercise routine at a mild to moderate level. However, if you have any doubts, always seek professional advice.

When to Avoid Exercise

Sometimes exercise is strictly forbidden to protect the health of the mother, the baby, or both. If you have any of the following conditions you will probably be advised not to exercise for the duration of your pregnancy:

- Pregnancy-induced hypertension (high blood pressure).
- Pre-term rupture of membranes (waters break too early).
- Pre-term labour, now or during previous pregnancy.
- Incompetent cervix (the end of the cervical canal opens much too early in the pregnancy).
- Persistent second or third trimester vaginal bleeding.
- Intrauterine growth retardation.
- Heart disease.
- Anaemia.
- Multiple pregnancy (twins or more).

TIPS

- Try this easy abdominal exercise: pull your clothes tight across your abdomen, tighten your abdominals and watch as your baby lifts up and in towards you. If your muscles are strong the degree of movement will amaze you.

- When bending down, keep your pelvis tilted and abdominals tight; bend from the knees and use your leg muscles to kneel down and stand up.

EXERCISE PLAN FOR PREGNANCY

During your first trimester, it is feasible for you to carry on as normal as long as you are feeling well and your doctor or healthcare professional permits it. Obvious exceptions are high-risk sports such as scuba diving and activities with a potential for hard falls such as horse-riding or water-skiing. Jogging and running fall into a grey area depending on whom you ask and therefore become a personal decision.

Some healthcare professionals see no reason for you to stop during your first (or even second) trimester, while others recommend curbing any impact activity (such as running and jumping). Fast walking, visits to the gym, aerobic classes and swimming are all safe options.

Abdominal exercises can be performed normally for the first 12 weeks, but after this avoid those that are done while lying on your back; see pages 120–121 for a few of the many safe variations.

WARNING SIGNS

If you have any of the following symptoms while you are exercising, stop immediately and contact your doctor or midwife:
• Pain anywhere, but especially in your back or pelvic region
• Excessive fatigue
• Dizziness
• Shortness of breath
• Feeling faint
• Vaginal bleeding
• Difficulty walking
• Contractions
• Unusual absence of foetal movements (but bear in mind that the baby is often most quiet when you are exercising)

EXERCISING AND BREASTFEEDING

Breastfeeding mothers should wear a good supporting bra and exercise after feeding the baby rather than before. This is to reduce the weight of the breasts and to avoid the loss of valuable nutrients due to leakage of milk from the nipples. Studies have shown that lactic acid levels (a by-product of exercise) in the milk increase following 30 minutes of aerobic activity. This increased lactic acid level was reported to give a bittersweet taste to the normally sweet milk, and the babies in the study were less likely to accept this.

GENERAL GUIDELINES

Don't go for the burn and exercise to exhaustion. Because you have less oxygen available for aerobic exercise, you should generally stick to 60 per cent of your maximum heart rate (MHR) while pregnant (see page 35). Your heart rate should not exceed 140 beats per minute.
• Slow down if you can't comfortably carry on a conversation.
• Make sure you stay cool during exercise, especially during the first trimester.
• Take frequent breaks and drink plenty of fluids.
• Avoid exercise in extremely hot weather, apart from swimming.
• Avoid contact sports during pregnancy.
• During the second and third trimesters, avoid any exercise that involves lying flat on your back as it can decrease the blood flow to your uterus.

Basic Pre-Natal Exercises

Try to do the following exercises 2–3 times a week. Remember to have a gentle warm-up before trying these exercises. Spend 5 minutes either walking at a medium pace or doing a combination of knee lifts, marching and leg curls (see pages 38–39). The pelvic floor exercises can be performed in any position – lying, standing or sitting – and can also be done secretly without it being obvious to anyone else around you, so try to do them as often as possible.

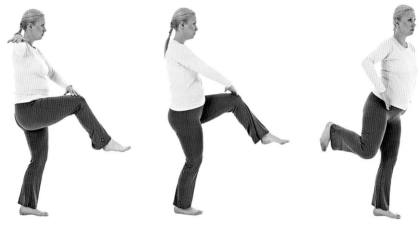

PELVIC FLOOR EXERCISES △

Slow Contractions
Stand, lie or sit with your feet slightly apart. Draw up and tighten the muscles around the anal sphincter; then hold. Slowly tighten the muscles around the urinary sphincter as well and lift up through the vagina. Hold for a count of 6, release with control and repeat.

4 x 4 reps

Fast Contractions
Stand, lie or sit with your feet slightly apart. Tighten all your pelvic floor muscles in one contraction. Hold for a count of 1, then release slowly.

4 x 6 reps

TECHNIQUE POINT
• If you have never worked these muscles, it may be difficult to isolate the movements individually, but it will get easier with practice.

KNEELING ABDOMINAL LIFT ▽

1 Kneel on all fours, with your hands directly beneath your shoulders, your fingers facing forwards and your knees under your hips. Keep your elbows soft. Let your abdomen relax but be careful not to let your back arch.

2 Breathe out and pull in your abdominals, lifting your baby in towards your spine. Keeping your elbows slightly bent, hold for a count of 6; remember to keep breathing throughout. Lower your abdominals under control and relax your abdomen.

2 x 8 reps

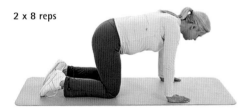

KNEELING ABDOMINAL CURL ▽

1 Kneel on all fours, with your hands directly beneath your shoulders, your fingers facing forwards and your knees under your hips. Keep your back and neck long and pull in the abdominals to prevent your back arching (see above).

2 Now tilt the pelvis and draw the baby up into you as you lift and round your back towards the ceiling. Keep breathing and hold for a count of 6. Gently lower until your back and neck are in line.

2 x 8 reps

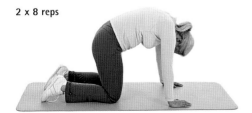

HIP HITCHES ▽

1 Kneel on all fours, with your hands directly beneath your shoulders, your fingers facing forwards and your knees under your hips. Keep your back and neck long and pull in the abdominals to prevent the back from arching.

2 Now, keeping the abdominals tight, draw your right hip up towards the right side of your ribcage keeping your upper body completely still. Return to centre and repeat the other way (you will feel like you are wiggling your buttocks).

2 x 8 reps

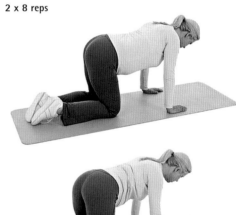

TECHNIQUE POINT
• Do not let the weight of your abdomen and breasts pull your back down, and arch your spine when you uncurl your body.

Getting Back in Shape

Deciding when to begin exercise after the birth of your baby is a very individual affair. Some mothers can't wait to get back into their pre-pregnancy clothes and, before long, will be following their old fitness regime. Others – probably the majority – have difficulty finding the time and motivation to get back into shape.

Whichever category you fall into, it is certainly advisable to undertake at least some basic exercise as soon as you feel up to it. With a new baby to care for, it can be difficult to make time to look after yourself, but the longer you put it off the harder it will be to get going and to shift that extra weight.

WHEN TO START?

However keen you are to get back into shape, you must wait until you have had the all-clear from your doctor. Normally this is 6 weeks after the birth for a natural birth and 12 weeks after a Caesarean. In the meantime, you may be given a sheet of simple exercises to follow for the first few weeks. These will include exercises like pelvic tilts, hip-hitching and head raises. Start with these, but remember that rest is vital at this time: take every opportunity to do so.

GETTING STARTED

Following your initial all-clear, it is still important to take things at a slower pace. The effect of the hormone relaxin (which helps the ligaments relax in preparation for childbirth) will put your joints as risk for 3–5 months following delivery. Consequently, this is not the right time to begin any form of exercise that requires great stability around the joints and especially the lumbar spine, such as weight training.

Because of this continued (although diminishing) effect of relaxin, all exercise should be performed with the utmost control and precision. Your posture will need retraining – remind yourself of this at every opportunity and refer to the five basic posture exercises (see pages 16–17).

DIASTASIS RECTI

The separation of your recti sheaths and resultant stretching of the linea alba (this is the fibrous union of the two sides of your abdominal muscles which stretches and separates to allow space for the growing baby) will gradually close over the first few weeks. While these are still separated in a condition known as diastasis recti, the abdominal muscles are unable to work efficiently. It is very important to check for diastasis before you resume normal abdominal, postural or lower-back exercises.

TEST FOR DIASTASIS ▽

1 Lie flat on your back, legs bent, and place your feet on the ground relatively close to your buttocks. Palms down, place 2 or 3 fingers below, on, or above the navel between the sheets of rectus abdominus. You may need to move your fingers around before you can be sure they are in the correct place.

2 Now pull in your abdominal muscles. Aiming to keep your stomach flat and pulled in (this may be quite difficult) raise your head off the floor, looking towards the tops of your toes.

The two sides of the rectus abdominus should close together on your fingers. If the gap is greater than 2 finger-widths wide, diastasis is still present. If so, only practise the static and pelvic tilts advised for the first six weeks after delivery (see page 124). As the separation decreases to 2 finger-widths, basic sit-ups may be introduced. If you are unsure about the condition of your abdominals, seek professional advice.

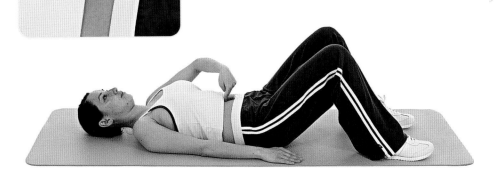

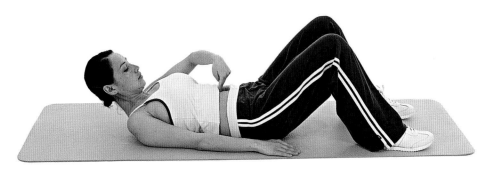

Post-Natal Exercises

Here are the exercises you are likely to be given to do for the first six weeks after labour. Make sure, however, that you get the all-clear from your midwife or doctor to do these and/or any other form of exercise.

How soon you can return to regular exercise will depend on your pre-pregnancy level of fitness, how much you exercised during pregnancy and how your body has coped with the pregnancy. As long as the abdominal muscles have returned to normal, you can progress with the resistance exercises. Any exercise that involves impact, such as jogging or the rebounder, should be attempted with caution. It is always best to consult a doctor before you get back into any form of exercising.

LYING PELVIC TILT ▽

1 Lie on your back with your knees bent and your feet flat on the floor, slightly less than hip-width apart. Relax your arms, either by your sides or resting gently on your stomach.

2 Lift your pubic bone gently upwards and feel the small of your back lightly touching the floor. Tighten your abdominal muscles and hold for a count of 6; keep breathing throughout. Release in a controlled way.

Gentle: 2 x 8 reps
Moderate: 2 x 16 reps
Energetic: 3 x 16 reps

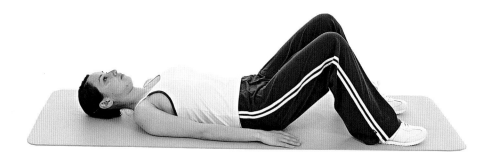

HEAD AND SHOULDER RAISE ▽

1 Lie on the floor with your knees bent and your feet flat on the floor, slightly less than hip-width apart. Place your hands on the base of your thighs, tilt your pelvis and tighten the abdominals.

2 Keeping your stomach firmly pulled in, breathe out and slowly raise your head, sliding your hands up towards your knees. Leave a space between your chin and chest as you lift. Lower yourself gently back down, breathing in as you do so. Keep your abdominal muscles tight and your pelvis tilted throughout.

Gentle: 2 x 8 reps
Moderate: 2 x 16 reps
Energetic: 3 x 16 reps

TECHNIQUE POINT
• Only raise your head and shoulders to a point where your abdominals can be held flat. If your stomach begins to push out (to 'dome'), make sure you keep the curl lower.

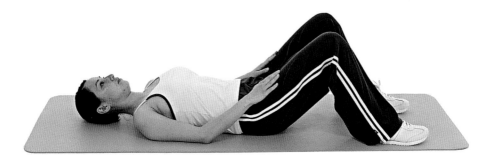

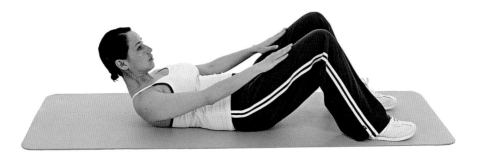

Index

Index / Acknowledgments

ACKNOWLEDGMENTS

All photography by **Octopus Publishing Group Ltd.**/
Peter Pugh-Cook except for the following:
Octopus Publishing Group Ltd./Stephen Conroy 24, 28
bottom centre left/ William Lingwood 28 bottom
/William Reavell 28 top centre, 28 centre/Simon Smith
26, 28 top/Karen Thomas 28 bottom centre right

Marks and Spencer plc, Baker Street, London W1
www.marksandspencer.com
Physical Company, High Wycombe, Buckinghamshire
HP12 1BG (0044) 01494-769222,
www.physicalcompany.co.uk

Models: **Rachel Clark** at Profile
also **Roger Magnus, Louisa Burgess** and
Anne-Marie Millard
Executive Editor: **Jane McIntosh**
Senior Editor: **Lisa John**
Editor: **Amy Corbett**
Executive Art Editor: **Mark Stevens**
Designer: **Ginny Zeal**
Illustrator: **Trevor Bounford**
Production Controller: **Manjit Sihra**